The Body You Want

The Body You Want

How to Epigenetically Combat Chronic Health Conditions

Dr. Christina Wachuku, PharmD.

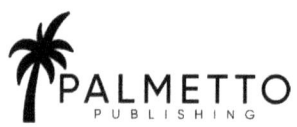

Charleston, SC

www.PalmettoPublishing.com

The Body You Want:
How to Epigenetically Combat Chronic Health Conditions

Copyright © 2022 by Dr. Christina Wachuku, PharmD

All rights reserved

No portion of this book may be reproduced, stored in a retrieval system, or transmitted in any form by any means–electronic, mechanical, photocopy, recording, or other–except for brief quotations in printed reviews, without prior permission of the author.

First Edition

Paperback ISBN: 978-1-63837-572-2
eBook ISBN: 978-1-63837-906-5

Disclaimer

While the author has taken utmost efforts to ensure the accuracy of the written content, all readers are advised to follow the information mentioned herein at their own risk. The author cannot be held responsible for any personal or commercial damage caused by misinterpretation of information. All readers are encouraged to seek professional advice when needed.

This book is for information purposes only. The author does not treat, diagnose, or claim to cure any disease. Every effort has been made to make this book as complete and accurate as possible. However, there may be mistakes in typography or content. Also, this book provides accurate information only up to the publishing date. Therefore, this book should be used as a guide and not as the ultimate source.

The purpose of this book is to educate. The author and the publisher do not claim that the information contained in this book is fully complete and shall not be responsible for any errors or omissions. The author and publisher shall have neither liability nor responsibility to any person or entity with respect to any loss or damage caused or alleged to be caused directly or indirectly by this book.

The information in this book is not intended to replace a one-on-one relationship with your primary care provider (PCP) or a qualified health care professional and is not intended as isolated medical advice. It is intended as a sharing of knowledge and information from the research and evidence of Christina Wachuku, PharmD, BCACP, ABAAHP, CMTM, CPH. Make the health care decisions that are right for you based on your research and in partnership with your PCP or qualified health care professional.

Table of Contents

Preface ix
Introduction 1
Chapter 1: Loneliness: An Unseen Killer .11
Chapter 2: How Childhood Trauma Impacts Health
    Across a Lifetime 19
Chapter 3: Role of Epigenetics in Parent-Child
    Transmission of Disease 25
Chapter 4: Are Epigenetic Changes Reversible? 31
Chapter 5: Your Health Matters 37
Chapter 6: The Power of Nutrition in Transforming Health 41
Chapter 7: Gut Health Issues Linked With Epigenetic Changes 49
Chapter 8: How To Choose the Right Nutritional Supplements 55
Chapter 9: Healthy Movement 61
Chapter 10: Restoring Sleep 65
Chapter 11: The Power of Your Thoughts 69
Conclusion 73
Acknowledgments 77
About the Author 79
References 81

Preface

The purpose of this book is to empower you with the knowledge that you can change the expression of your genes within your lifetime and future generations.

Since epigenetic changes are reversible, you can combat the development of diseases by changing your lifestyle and eating habits. You don't have to stay sick or suffer from health issues for the rest of your life. You can make the choice to control your own health, and it all begins in the mind. So mind your thoughts.

Introduction

Our genes are not our destiny! What we do and what happens to us matter. We can turn off bad genes and turn on good ones by changing what we eat, what we think about, how much we sleep, how well we are paying attention to our nutritional deficiencies, and how well we move our bodies. Our genes don't change, but our gene behaviors do!

This book will teach you how to be more aware of what your body want by learning how your body functions and how to pay close attention to what your body is saying and take prompt action to fix the underlying problems. Lifestyle Disease does not come without a cause. Unresolved emotional trauma and stress, including negative thoughts can influence our health in a profound way. Some other underlying causes of disease are the environmental stresses that overwhelm the body's ability to maintain balance. These include nutritional deficiencies, toxic overload and mental and emotional stress such as marital problems, toxic relationships, negative work environment and other life situations.

You don't just wake up and become chronic all of a sudden. Every modern lifestyle chronic disease state starts out as an acute process then progresses to a chronic disease state when you violate the 8 laws of health (Nutrition, Exercise, water, sunlight, temperance, fresh air, proper rest, and trust in God.). When you repeatedly abuse your body and neglect the signs your body is telling you to see, then there's a cascade of events that will start off the disease process through imbalances in tissue state and each stage progresses slowly in a predictable way. Prompt intervention at any of the stages is likely to be more effective if the root cause is stopped than treatment given after the disease has progressed and become symptomatic. Praise the Lord for second chances. Just like the lifestyle disease process is progressive, it is also reversible and can be prevented with healthy lifestyle changes. It is so comforting and healing to know that with the right knowledge, you can take steps to interrupt the progression of early adversity to disease and prevent chronic health issues later in life. You can reverse the process. Every disease starts with irritation which may presents as inflammation. The subacute stage is the transitional phase between the acute and the chronic stages. If not treated, the inflammation will result in pain, the body's most effective warning sign. If no intervention is rendered, then it progresses to a chronic state of disease which is the slowing down of the body's operation. This chronic state can last for months to even years and then eventually results in a degenerative disease state.

Chronic diseases are not cured when you take medications, you are only managing the disease state or multiple chronic disease states. You may be able to suppress specific symptoms with drugs or remove diseased tissue with surgery but unfortunately, the root causes are still unresolved. The underlying problems are still going on. This is because the symptoms are the results, not the root cause of the disease. When you gain understanding of how chronic disease happen, you are well informed and empowered with the knowledge to fix the underlying problems.

Health and chronic disease depend on how you choose to treat your body. When your body is complaining with the symptoms presented, you should learn how to listen and take action. This is the body's attempt to get rid of the irritants. You can choose to learn how your body function so that you can know how to remove stressors and support weak body systems to allow the body to heal itself. If you choose to follow the eight Principles of Health and make the necessary dietary and lifestyle changes, the body will have enough strength to get itself back to harmony.

When you learn to reduce stress, minimize your daily exposure to environmental toxins, heal unresolved emotional conflicts, forgive and let go of the past traumas, adopt a positive mental attitude, maintain supportive social connections, fix your digestive problems, take appropriate nutritional supplements daily and live a healthy lifestyle, you will be able to combat chronic disease and have the body we want.

Epigenetics is the study of changing how a gene behaves without changing the gene itself.

There are strong links between epigenetics and chronic disease, showing that life experiences can trigger our risks for specific chronic conditions.

The US National Center for Health Statistics defines chronic disease as a condition lasting for three months or more. About half of all adults suffer from a chronic condition, and a third of the population has multiple conditions that limit their usual activity.

More than 75 percent of all health care costs are due to chronic conditions. By the year 2023, it is projected that people in the United States will spend $4.2 trillion in treatment costs. National health spending is projected to grow at an average annual rate of 5.5 percent for 2019–28 and to reach $6.2 trillion by 2028. If you think staying healthy is kind of expensive, getting sick is so much more expensive!

If one person is sick in the house with a chronic condition or an infection, the quality of life of all family members can be affected. This may lead to sacrifices such as taking time off from work to care for the sick family member, cancelling social events to stay home with the sick child, spending savings to pay for medical expenses, and worrying constantly about the lack of improvement in their health conditions.

Improving our immune system is of utmost importance for everyone. It is a good idea to take a multivitamin every day. Eat a well-balanced diet. Get at least eight hours of sleep every night. Drink plenty of water.

Remember, the best way to build up your immune system and overall health includes the eight NEWSTART Lifestyle Program principles: nutrition, exercise, water, sunlight, temperance, fresh air, proper rest, and trust in God. NEWSTART is a physician-monitored, scientifically researched lifestyle change program to prevent and reverse disease through natural methods. Examples of how to support your health using nutritional supplements to naturally boost your immune system for a healthier lifestyle include taking Isotonix Vitamin D with K2, Isotonix Immune, Isotonix Vitamin C, Isotonix Daily Essentials Packets, Isotonix OPC, etc.

These are isotonic formulations that enter the digestive tract in liquefied form and supply nutrients at just the right rate to your body. This eliminates the need for further breakdown in the stomach with maximum absorption, compared to retail-sold tablet formulation vitamins. They are only available through a health care provider.

There was a ten-year-old girl who was born in New York City but grew up in Nigeria, who loved family vacations and long-distance trips. She enjoyed the rest stops along the way and especially the ones at restaurants and busy intersections where salespeople run to cars to sell snacks and drinks to travelers. At this tender age, she didn't care that the Nigerian roads were full of potholes, that there were no streetlights, and that people were always speeding. She just loved the journey.

One day, this little girl and her family got on the road and embarked on another long journey. Most of her siblings were asleep in the back seat, and her parents took turns driving, keeping themselves awake via good conversation and laughter.

Suddenly, the clouds started to roll in, and the sky started to get darker. Rain started to pour, thunder roared, and lightning struck across the sky, as if in anger. It was then that it all happened.

An eighteen-wheeler trailer ahead of them suddenly lost balance and collided with a brown Volvo SUV in the narrow oncoming lane. The Volvo somersaulted and flipped six times before landing upside down.

The trailer continued its path of destruction, a moving monster that hit multiple cars before it could be stopped. What had started out as a fun family vacation had turned into a horror show.

The little girl's family was safe, and they pulled off to the side of the road, but all the girl could do was cry. That little girl was me.

As I grew into my teenage years, I became increasingly anxious whenever we went on long trips. They weren't fun anymore, and my heart raced anytime we took a trip. I constantly looked over my shoulders and kept checking for trailers on the road. I hated how they sped past us, hated the deafening sound and their frightening size. I sat on the edge of my seat whenever I saw one fast approaching from behind and would beg my dad to please hurry up and drive faster, so the trailer wouldn't catch up with us. I would shut my eyes tight, not wanting to relive that horrible trip.

Long trips became my least favorite adventures, and when it came time for me to learn how to drive, I came up with excuses as to why I couldn't. I had come to associate driving with dying.

After high school, my dad renewed our US passports. We moved back to New York, and I enrolled in college. My dad signed me up for driving lessons even though I really didn't want to get behind the wheel of a car. When I finally got my driver's license, I refused to buy a car. After all, buying a car meant driving a car, and the streets in NYC were always so crowded. Plus, parking was always a problem in the city, so I did not see the point. I had witnessed people fighting for alternate parking spots and unending tickets being issued to drivers every day, and I didn't want to get involved in that struggle.

I tried to take the city subway everywhere I went. I relocated to Florida for a career growth opportunity and was compelled to drive. Not having the convenience of trains readily available and the fact that everything was so far apart made driving a necessity. In fact, my job was over fifty miles away from my house. Because of this, I bought a car, and I reluctantly started driving.

I soon realized that my anxiety from that first traumatic event had never left me; it had just gotten buried deep in my subconscious mind. Even to this day, I'm always alert and ready, seldom relaxed while sitting in the driver's seat. I always look straight ahead, keeping my eyes 100 percent on the road, even when I have an active companion in the passenger seat. I never look down to get my phone or eat or drink, and I always stay within the speed limit for safety purposes.

I am not just a pharmacist; I am also a patient. I remember the day at the doctor's office when I was told I have high blood pressure (BP), right after my first car accident, which had taken place just five minutes from my house at a busy intersection. When the doctor told me that, I was frustrated. *Why me?* I thought, *Why now?* As a pharmacist, I already knew a lot about health and wellness and chronic disease. I knew about disease prevention, and I knew most chronic conditions have a cause; they do not usually happen randomly or overnight. My family has a history of hypertension, so I had been careful to eat well and keep an eye on my own blood pressure. When I found out I had high blood pressure, I wondered if my traumatic childhood experience and the resulting anxiety throughout the rest of my life contributed to it.

According to the most recent guidelines, normal blood pressure is 120/80 mm Hg or less. Hypertension is when blood pressure is greater than

130/80 mm Hg. It is worth noting that one high reading does not mean you have chronically high blood pressure. It is necessary to measure your blood pressure at different times while you are resting comfortably for at least five minutes. To be diagnosed with hypertension, at least three elevated blood pressure readings are required at least one week apart.

I was started on a blood pressure medication called hydrochlorothiazide, commonly known as a water pill. Upon my follow-up visit, my doctor added another blood pressure medication, lisinopril.

After about six months into my regimen, my lips started swelling up suddenly and at random times. It was embarrassing because it could happen anywhere and at any time. It started with a numb feeling as I was driving to work, and then my lips were noticeably swollen within the hour. If it happened at work, I had to get permission from my pharmacy supervisor to see the nurse practitioner in the same building as the pharmacy I worked at. The first time this happened, I asked what she thought the cause might be. She said I was obviously allergic to something—it could be anything from using a new soap to a new body lotion to eating something I wasn't used to. I wasn't happy with her answer because I was hoping she'd be able to just take a look at my lips and tell me what had caused the swelling and how to stop it.

A few months later, it happened again while I was driving. I was seen by the same nurse practitioner and asked her if my lisinopril could be the culprit since I was only on those two drugs. She said no—it wasn't possible since I'd been on the drug for at least six months at that point. I wasn't satisfied with her answer and started researching more. As a pharmacist, I already knew that lisinopril had an uncommon side effect called angioedema—swelling of the lips, tongue, and face—and this happens in less than one in one hundred people. The only problem with the theory is that, as the nurse practitioner had said, I had been on it for many months with no side effects and never developed a cough, which is usually the more common side effect. Although uncommon, angioedema can occur late in therapy, and it can actually appear six to ten years after treatment—even if there were no symptoms before then. I was determined to get to the bottom of this and asked my primary care physician to change my lisinopril to another safer alternative, just in case. I was switched to another class of an antihypertensive drug called a beta-blocker, and I was prescribed metoprolol. I was relieved and was sure my days of swollen lips were over.

As I returned to my PCP for subsequent visits, I was told again and again that my blood pressure was still too high. I was disappointed because I had been following the plan closely and hadn't had any problems with the new drug. I started wondering what more I could do since I was still young and didn't want to be on medication for the rest of my life. I cut down on my salt intake, started exercising more, and even lost weight, but nothing seemed to work. I bought a blood pressure monitor and started keeping a record to take to my PCP's office. My blood pressure readings were always high, in the 140s/90s, the same range as in the doctor's office.

I began to do more research at home and became interested in pharmacogenomics (PGx) and gene single nucleotide polymorphism (SNP) DNA analysis-precision medicine. I took a certification exam in this subject, which is designed to teach pharmacists how to integrate pharmacogenomics into practice to improve medication use and show people how to choose the right medicine from the start. Pharmacogenomics is about choosing safer medicine the first time instead of the standard trial and error method of matching patients with medication.

Using the PGx test, doctors can use a patient's genetic profile and prescribe the best available medicine right from the start, every time. I was excited and decided to order my own PGx test. The company I partnered with sent me a DNA collection kit that used a noninvasive mouth swab. When I got the results back, I was surprised. I found out that I was a CYP2D6 Ultra Metabolizer, which means that my gene variation was increasing the conversion of metoprolol into inactive metabolites. Because of this, my doctor should increase my dosage even though doing so may increase the side effects. The amount of metoprolol I was taking was insufficient for me even though I was already taking the maximum recommended dose. What this means is I was not metabolizing metoprolol correctly and, therefore, I wasn't getting the therapeutic effect and was just wasting my time and money. I sent a summary copy of my PGx result to my physician and asked him to switch me to an alternative drug. He accepted my recommendation and switched me to bisoprolol, and I noticed an improvement in my BP readings at home the very next day. When I went back to the clinic with my logbook, my doctor was impressed! He took my BP in his office, and it was good: 100/70 mm Hg. I started eating more green leafy veggies and cruciferous vegetables to naturally lower my blood pressure. I made sure my main dish includes a salad and filled up my plate with 7 to 10 cups of vegetables everyday including kale, spinach, celery, broccoli, okra, cabbage, collard green, cauliflower, watercress etc. I would mix bell pepper, onion, tomatoes, and spinach into my morning egg omelet. I would eat fresh fruits such as the triple berries and bananas for dessert or make a smoothie, my favorite being blueberries, raspberries and strawberries. I would also add varieties of fresh vegetables to make soups.

Moreover, I was intentional by deliberately setting my phone alarm clock to remind me to drink a glass of water every hour. I vary the intake to 8–12 glasses of water per day purposefully and avoid drinking water right before and after meals for an hour. Thanks be to God, the giver of water and life.

I continued to change my lifestyle habits and began walking thirty minutes every day while watching my weight by eating healthy meals. I also began taking nutritional supplements, including omega-3 fatty acid and coenzyme Q10.

A year later, my blood pressure was 94/60 mm Hg and stayed consistently within that range. I decided to work with my physician to cut back on my dose with the goal of weaning off my medications. These days, I continue to check my BP readings even though my blood pressure has successfully returned to normal. More importantly, I pay attention to living a healthy lifestyle to keep my blood pressure low.

I chose to attempt to lower my blood pressure by investing in personalized medicine to gain insight into identifying my own unique gene variations and solving the underlying problem. I was able to change my diet and lifestyle to help promote optimal health. I did it, and so can you.

The purpose of this book is to empower you to ask your health care providers more questions about your health and do your own research until you get the answers you're looking for. The goal is for every patient to become an active participant in their own care. Learn how to listen to the messages your body is sending you to prevent sickness. Say yes to self-care and know that you have the choice to live a healthier lifestyle and gain the confidence to write your own prescription of wellness in creating your own reality. Learn how to revitalize your body's innate ability to reverse your chronic conditions. So let's get started!

chapter 1

Loneliness: An Unseen Killer

Are you capable of making friends? You are certainly not incapable of making friends, but to have a real friend, you must be a friend through good and bad times. Don't be too hard on yourself. This chapter will show you what habits can help you build good, solid friendships for the long term.

Loneliness is a state of mind and has become a disease in itself. It is a major problem, especially for the elderly. According to a research study at the University of California, San Francisco, over 40 percent of people over age sixty regularly suffer from intense loneliness. Loneliness can have a serious impact on health and well-being, and scientists are beginning to see the seriousness of the damage that chronic loneliness can cause. According to the Association for Psychological Science, it is as damaging as smoking fifteen cigarettes a day, is as detrimental to health as obesity, and can increase the premature death rate by 26 percent.

One landmark study shows that social isolation is correlated with high blood pressure and obesity.

Recent research into epigenetics shows how genes are expressed and how they can be adversely affected, impairing the body's ability to turn off inflammation. Chronic inflammation has been linked to heart disease, arthritis, type 2 diabetes, cancer, Alzheimer's disease, and even suicide attempts.

A sociological research study revealed that over 25 percent of Americans do not have a close friend to confide in.

Each of us has the innate desire for emotional intimacy with others, and this intimacy is important for our development as human beings. We love being acknowledged by other people, being able to fit in with our peers, and interacting with friends and loved ones. We also have times when we prefer to be in our own space to self-reflect and be creative. Together, these create a healthy balance. The problem begins when we cannot find a balance between belonging and solitude. How have you been affected by the Covid-19 pandemic?

Joy is a fifteen-year-old teenager who was told by her family that they would have to relocate out of state due to her dad's job promotion. When they told her, she suddenly became very quiet and went to her room. Later, her mom came in to check on her and found her crying. When her mom asked why she was crying, Joy responded, "Why do we always have to uproot our whole lives and move? I will never see my friends again!" Her mom watched in astonishment as her crying became more hysterical and her anger more explosive.

At her new school, Joy found it increasingly difficult to make new friends. She would keep a serious face in class and walked past other students every day for weeks, waiting for them to make the first move. She wasn't proud or pompous; she just found it impossible to take a chance and say something first for fear of rejection. She didn't speak during class and became known as the quietest girl in school. She had no friends and felt paralyzed with fear. It seemed as though everyone just ignored her. When she asked a question in class, everyone made fun of her. When she ate in the cafeteria, nobody joined her table, and she always ended up eating all alone.

In her biology class, students often worked in groups. When the teacher asked the class who would like to work with Joy, there was an awkward silence until, eventually, the teacher paired her up with a group.

Joy felt constantly rejected, and this dampened her self-esteem. She felt awful every morning getting ready for school. She felt so bored and alone, even among her peers. She was constantly being bullied and made fun of. She wanted to quit school.

The feeling of emptiness began to follow her home. Her family members were always on their phones, even at dinnertime, including Joy. Communication between them was lost. Joy had social skills, but she was still missing those important deeper connections. She eventually reached out to her dad and told him she's had enough. She was tired of not having a close friend to confide in. She was tired of only having superficial relationships. Her dad encouraged her to stop holding on to her past and to focus on the present. She eventually had to train her mind to stop living in the past, where she had lots of good friends. She trained her mind to stop playing the "if" game and start living in the present moment, living in her own truth. Once she let go of the past, she began to smile and talk to fellow students instead of using her phone as her relational crutch whenever she felt insecure. She joined her high school dance team where she felt exhilarated. After all, there is strength in vulnerability and being vulnerable connects us with others.

Internet addiction disorder has recently been added to the *Diagnostic and Statistical Manual of Mental Disorders* as a disorder that needs more research.

Are you suffering from this disorder? Do you spend extreme amounts of time playing video games on the internet? Do you compulsively shop online? Are you constantly checking your Facebook account? Is your excessive computer use interfering with your relationships, work, or school? Do you constantly check your phone every time a text comes through? If you answer yes to any of these questions, you are not alone. The internet itself isn't negative, but just like anything else, we need balance. Spending too much time on social media can have unintended side effects, such as sitting for long periods of time and spending too much time in isolation away from your loved ones. Needless to say, social media platforms like Facebook, Instagram, and Snapchat have been shown to increase the risks for depression and loneliness.

Dan Buettner, a *National Geographic* writer, took a special look at the Blue Zones—places with a high concentration of people who live past ninety years old without chronic diseases. Buettner states that loneliness can shave eight years off your life expectancy. What an unseen killer loneliness is!

He also mentions that Seventh-day Adventists, especially those living in Loma Linda, have a strong face-to-face social network where they frequently do things together. These activities include attending church, hiking, and hosting potlucks. These kinds of gatherings are enormously powerful but vastly undercelebrated. Buettner concludes that if social connectedness and volunteerism were pharmaceuticals, they would be blockbuster drugs.

Epigenetics makes us unique. We have different personalities. Some people are outspoken while some are shy. Some are sociable while some are not. We all have different fingerprints and genetic variations that make us who we are. We differ from one another, from our gender to our eye colors, to the types of food that work best with our bodies, to the types of exercise designed to make each of us perform optimally. We are all unique, and you can't blend in when you were born to stand out. Be proud of your unique qualities and be comfortable in your own skin.

Here are some practical solutions to combat loneliness:

Talk to someone about your loneliness. Someone once said, "Divine power is not summoned to do what human power can do." Ask for help. Just say, "I think I'm lonely." Most people would like to help if only you would ask. But if you don't ask, they'll assume you're fine. Let go of your insecurities and your ego. Humble yourself and take that first step of asking for help. Look inward anytime you feel lonely. The power to change how you feel in the moment is right inside of you. Give yourself permission to be happy by not depending on others for your own happiness. Practice self-acceptance by embracing what makes you unique. Every time you feel sad, do some talk therapy. Say to yourself, "I am enough for me."

Be thankful for the problems you don't have, such as the problem of dealing with gossip and backbiting that can come from having too many friends.

Start by making yourself vulnerable. Be your authentic self. For instance, if you are asked to talk in a group and you feel nervous, go ahead and say you are feeling nervous. Not only will this confession help you relax, but it will also make others feel better about their own imperfections and allow them to better relate with you.

Start by gradually building rapport with people. Make small talk. Say "hi" to strangers. Ask someone what their name is, compliment their hairstyle, ask where they got it done. If you like to cook, let them know and ask if they like it as well. It doesn't matter what you make small talk about. The purpose is to create connections and rapport.

Distract yourself by becoming busy. Get a journal and start writing how you want to feel. There is power in positive thinking. Use your imagination to escape to a wonderland in your mind as often as you want. Whenever you feel lonely, take a trip back to where you feel happy and connected in your mind. Connect with anyone you wish to inside your mind.

Read more books. Challenge your negative thoughts. Do something creative when you are alone. Learn how to love yourself through daily self-care. Work on reducing your stress levels. Take deep breaths and relax more often.

Restrict time spent on social media to two hours per day by setting a timer on your phone or on social media app..

Volunteer your time to help others and give back. Show an act of kindness to someone new every day. Give someone your time. Mentor a kid in your community. Volunteer your time at your local library to help seniors learn to use a computer. Support your church by actively participating in community events. Share your money or resources with the homeless. Helping someone else will give you a sense of purpose and make you feel happy in the moment. Be present every moment of the day. Yes, you can do it.

Find a support group or social club in your area via resources such as Meetup.com and be an active participant. Tell them your story and show interest in theirs.

Choose to invest in a life coach. We all need people in our lives to help us move toward positive changes. Find a coach to guide and support you to reduce the power of emotional tension.

I'll leave it to your discretion and due diligence to consider signing up as an Airbnb location if you live alone. My family once booked a vacation at a big house where a retired woman lived alone. She shared the story of how her ex-husband was a pedophile, and she divorced him. She told us all her children were grown and have their own lives and, therefore, she was left alone with this empty house. She had a disability that prevented her from working, so she decided to take action and do something about her situation. She made a decision to work on her garden every morning and use her extra rooms for Airbnb to make some income.

She generously provided breakfast for her visitors and made herself available for questions and social interaction. We learned so much from her, and she indeed made our stay memorable. She had a sense of purpose to make the world a better place.

If you are religious, spend time in prayer and reading the Bible. Believe and you will receive. Prayer can help you come to realizations that you might not have seen before. Imagine you are far from home in a dark building you aren't familiar with, and you need to use the restroom. You know the restroom is on the other side of the wall in front of you, but you can't find a way through. If you could only just walk a few steps to the right, you would've seen there's an open passageway, but you could not see it in the darkness. And so you pound on the wall, trying in vain to get it to break. The solution is only a few feet away from you, but you can't see it. When you pray, the thought might pop into your head to walk to the right and see what happens. In doing so, you find the passage through the wall. A word of prayer is all that is needed to give you the strength and the courage to take that step in the right direction. If you are struggling with pain, anger, and loneliness, pray for strength. It is on our knees that we fight the hardest battles.

You have the choice to choose to pray and believe that you will receive. And you will receive. God can hear your breaking heart, your loneliness, your fear, and your frustration. You don't need a lot of fake friends; you only need a few good ones that you can depend on. Ask God to help you meet three good friends that you can confide in, and you will receive. Remember that you are never truly alone.

Several other effective methods to combat loneliness are to combine exercise and socialization by joining a yoga class, a walking group, or a gym. Pets can also reduce loneliness by providing companionship.

Loneliness has become a public health concern because research shows that intense loneliness can increase health problems. It can cause you aches, sadness, pain, depression, suicidal ideation, increased stress levels, poor decision-making, and increased risk of heart problems and stroke, just to name a few.

In 2011, Bronnie Ware published the book *The Top Five Regrets of the Dying*, which compiled the regrets her dying patients confessed having. According to her findings, most people wished they had kept in touch more with friends who mattered.

Some people are meant to stay in your life only for a season, some old friends or even family members are meant to be loved from a distance and it's a good idea to let go of toxic relationships but if you have good friends that you've lost touch with, take action today as tomorrow is not promised. Send a simple text, make a phone call, connect with them through social media. Be bold and make the first move. Have no regrets.

The truth is that good friendships do take efforts. The good news is it is not too late for you to reconnect. Stop putting it off till tomorrow, pick up the phone, apologize if you have to and start restoring those friendships that matter.

A research study from the University of California, Los Angeles, shows that people with strong social interactions have a stronger gene expression for immunity, which is a key to optimal health.

As you strive to continue to improve your health, remember how important it is to also have strong social interactions. If you are feeling lonely and don't have anyone to connect with, remember you can always choose to connect with God from within your heart and stay blessed.

Mother Teresa said, "The greatest disease in the West today is not tuberculosis or leprosy; it is being unwanted, unloved, and uncared for. While we can cure physical disease by taking medication, the only prescription to cure loneliness is love."

Smile first. Make the first move to shake hands. Say "hi" first. Hug someone first. Give compliments first. Show empathy. Give a listening ear. Offer your support and encouragement. Invite someone for dinner. Offer to pray with someone. Express your feelings and let that person know that you care. Let's all do our part to make this world a better place. You can start by loving your neighbor as yourself and do unto others as you would have them do unto you.

chapter two

How Childhood Trauma Impacts Health Across a Lifetime

Mike was the fifth child out of seven. He grew up in a beautiful part of town with big houses and lots of trees and blooming flowers. His father worked in construction and was responsible for the building of many gorgeous houses. His mother, young and beautiful, was the head principal of a top-performing high school in town.

His dad was well known in the city as the most generous, understanding man you'd ever meet. He was the guy who would stand up for what is right, no matter what. He used to help the less fortunate people in the neighborhood who had nothing to eat and nowhere to sleep. He'd invite them home and would feed them time and time again. He was a strict but fair parent, and everyone loved him. He was healthy and vibrant and never stepped into the hospital a day in his life.

One cold night, Mike found out his dad was ill. Something that just started out as a cough grew overnight into body aches and a high fever, and he was rushed to the hospital. Things took a turn for the worse, and within days, at the young age of forty-eight, Mike's father died. The whole town wept bitterly, and Mike, just twelve years old at the time, was deeply affected.

His mom, now left with seven young, active children, was beside herself and did not know how to keep on living. She quickly slipped into depression and developed mental health issues. She lost the will to live and couldn't function. She quit her job and would cry for days at a time. Suddenly, in her early forties, she had a stroke. Mike was left to take care of his mom while all the older siblings were away at college. Most days, he would skip school to make sure his mom took her medication and ate the right foods. Unfortunately, as much as Mike tried to nurture his mom back to health, all she wanted to do was give up. She couldn't live life without her soul mate. She would cry and ask, "Why did you do this to me, honey?" over and over again.

One day, when Mike once again had to take the day off from school to look after his mom, he found some of his mother's medication under the bedsheet where she had hidden them and realized she had stopped taking her medication. He also discovered that every time he left for school, she would indulge in all the wrong foods the doctor had warned her to stop eating, such as ice cream, cakes, cookies, and chocolate bars. Suddenly, her facial expression changed, she drooled, her speech slurred, her muscles stiffened, and the left side of her body went numb. Mike was frightened by this sudden change and was rightfully angry with her. Unfortunately, his mom did not make it past that day. She died exactly three years after her husband. She resolved to share his fate, choosing to die with him rather than to live without him. Mike was just fifteen at the time. After a person experiences a stroke, the likelihood of having another is significant within the first five years.

Mike and his siblings had to be separated and divided among close relatives, some as far from each other as one thousand miles.

Many days ahead were rough. Mike was neglected and mistreated by his relatives and went days without food. He was used as a house boy and had to miss many days of schoolwork due to the nonpayment of his tuition. While his friends at school began to talk about what they wanted to be when they grew up, Mike was lost and could only think about how to survive the days ahead. When he complained at home about being treated unfairly, he was sent packing to his other uncle's house. The poor treatment continued everywhere he went. Everyone favored their own children over him, and he grew bitter, remembering how his own dad had treated everyone equally. He became rebellious and disobedient and, as a result, was punished frequently.

One day, Mike decided he'd had enough. He gathered all he had and left without letting anyone know where he was going. Many nights, he slept in empty classrooms, arranging the desks to lay on them for the night. Some nights, Mike found himself sneaking into an abandoned construction site. Other nights, he just slept on the roadside. He was living on the streets in the most dangerous part of the city.

He made bad decisions and started engaging in high-risk behaviors. He got in with a bad crowd and started smoking, doing drugs, and sleeping with whoever he wanted.

A few years later, Mike got the horrifying news that his younger brother, John had been in a fight with bullies at school and was badly injured. John had a direct contact with an infected person who was coughing and sneezing while bullying him. John was taken to the local hospital and diagnosed with meningitis. He took ill and was soon pronounced dead. Three deaths in the family, one right after another.

To cope, Mike got more involved with nightclubs, violence, and women. There seemed to be no turning back.

One day, he was cornered by gang members and was robbed and beaten at gunpoint. He was beaten so badly that his friends couldn't recognize him. He was attacked because he had been found dancing with a beautiful girl who happened to be dating one of the most notorious gang members. He was lucky to escape with his life.

One of his uncles who was in California heard about this and decided to enroll him into a private Christian university where his life was forever changed for good. He had no choice but to make friends with people who loved the Lord. He was invited to their homes when school was out and made close relationships. They became his family. After all, the true meaning of family is people who support and love you, people you can trust and confide in, regardless of whether you are related. He lives to tell his story today. What a testimony it is when you choose to turn your life around. You have the freedom of choice—always remember that.

According to the Centers for Disease Control and Prevention (CDC), adverse childhood experiences, or ACEs, are potentially traumatic events that occur during childhood (birth to seventeen years). They include experiencing violence, abuse, or neglect; witnessing violence in the home; or having a family member attempt or die by suicide. Also included are aspects of the child's environment that can undermine their sense of safety, stability, and bonding such as growing up in a household with substance abuse, mental health problems, instability due to parental separation, or incarceration of a parent, sibling, or another member of the household.

Traumatic events in childhood can be emotionally painful or distressing and can have effects that persist for years.

When ACEs are intense or numerous, they can affect brain development, the immune system, and the hormonal system; can trigger epigenetic changes that increase the risk of mental illness and poor educational achievements; and can lead to chronic disease. These chronic diseases include obesity, diabetes, depression, suicide attempts, sexually transmitted disease, heart disease, cancer, stroke, and Chronic obstructive pulmonary disease and the lists goes on.

Adverse childhood experiences and their effects are things everybody needs to know about.

A study was conducted where 17,500 adults were asked about the history of exposure to a toxic childhood environment, and for every "yes" a score was assigned. The score was then compared to health outcomes, and the results were astonishing. They found that ACEs are incredibly common and that there was a dose-response relationship between ACEs and health outcomes. This means that the higher you score, the worse your health outcome.

Children are sensitive to the effects of repeated stress activation when their brains and bodies are still developing. This massive dose of repeated stress can affect brain structure and how the brain functions; it can affect the immune system and trigger epigenetic changes that are frequently long-lasting and can lead to disease. Thankfully, these epigenetic changes are also reversible.

Imagine you get a flat tire on a long journey when it is starting to get dark. You quickly pull over and try to change the damaged tire. Suddenly, a big white van pulls over a few blocks ahead of you, and you're glad somebody is going to help you out. To your surprise, two heavily built men climb out of the van with guns and proceed toward you. Immediately, your hypothalamus sends a signal to your pituitary, which sends a signal to your adrenal glands to change gear for an immediate rescue mission. Stress hormones are released. Adrenaline and cortisol come to the rescue. You can hear your heart pounding, and you run as fast as you can into the dark bushes. This stress response is a perfect reaction to save your life.

The problem is that if these two heavily built men with guns were to continue to show up every day where you park your car, or if the vivid memory of them plays every time you park, it would activate your fight-or-flight response system repeatedly. This life-saving mechanism can then damage your health, and the effects of it may persist to the next generation.

Do you suffer from or know of a family member who suffers from mental health issues? Do you have an alcoholic parent, or have you experienced domestic abuse? This is an ongoing issue that touches all of us, and the repercussions can continue affecting us long after the danger has passed. Learning how to tell your story and taking steps to interrupt the progression of early adversity to disease are crucial to preventing chronic health issues later in life.

To help reduce the number of ACEs, first ensure a strong start for your children. Promote safe dating and healthy relationships. Strengthen household financial security such as tax credits or childcare assistance. Connect youth to after-school programs such as the Boys & Girls Club or YMCA (The Y). Do not let your children be exposed to violence at home. Be a positive role model for them. Teach your children how to handle stress and manage their emotions. If you have children that are currently being affected, refer them promptly to mental health services. Enroll them in mentoring programs that support children through difficulties.

If you notice someone you love is engaging in dangerous and illegal activities, tell authorities and get them the help they need. Engage in shared responsibility for the health and well-being of all children. Treat symptoms to lessen the harms of ACEs. Practice holistic interventions such as thirty minutes of daily mindfulness. Mindfulness is basically living in the moment with kindness and awareness. You can engage in mindful activities such as yoga, mindful eating, and learning to breathe. These interventions are designed to help build awareness, creativity, and imagination while being fully present in the moment.

If you have been a victim, you can choose to start writing down the stories of what happened to you. Writing down your deepest emotions continuously for twenty minutes every day can have positive health effects. Remember, you have the power to decide to later burn the paper or destroy the written pages.

Just the act of venting your anger is healing instead of keeping those hurtful emotions boiled up inside of you. Let it all out on paper. Make the decision to seek professional help by going to therapy and consider medication if necessary. You have the power to choose healthy diets and nutritional supplements to boost your immune system.

Remember, ACEs and their associated harms are preventable, treatable, and beatable, but it's going to take all of us banding together to help each other.

chapter three

Role of Epigenetics in Parent-Child Transmission of Disease

The outside environment has effects on our genes that can influence the development of a disease, and some of these effects are inherited. They can even be passed on to future generations.

Recent reports predict that by 2030, half of all adults in the United States will be obese.

Combating chronic disease requires reversing negative environmental factors, and epigenetics holds the key. Before we continue, let's look a little deeper into what epigenetics is.

Epigenetics is the study of how lifestyle and the environment influence the expression of genes and how these changes can be passed on to the next generation. In other words, epigenetics controls genes. The genetic code you get from your mother and father determines many things about you. The genes you inherit are made up of DNA code that was set before you were born. While in utero, your genes were very sensitive and changeable, according to things such as your mother's stress, what she ate, where she lived, when she slept, how well she exercised, her thought processes, and whom she interacted with. While these genes were set before you were born, you can alter them now, and that can change how you grow for the rest of your life. Since many diseases, such as obesity, diabetes, heart disease, and cancer, and mental illnesses are influenced by epigenetic mechanisms, epigenetic drugs offer a potential way to reverse abnormal gene expression that can lead to disease progression.

There was a study done in northern Sweden to determine whether nutrition affects death rates caused by heart disease and diabetes. It also looked at whether these effects could be passed on from parents to their children and grandchildren.

They examined the availability of food according to records of yearly harvest, as well as food prices across three generations in northern Sweden.

Data was collected from the years 1890, 1905, and 1920. The researchers found that if food was not readily available during the father's slow growth period due to famine, his sons were less likely to die from heart disease. Slow growth period in midchildhood is defined as a sensitive time before the start of puberty when environmental factors have the most impact on body development. This period right before puberty is critical to determining whether their genes will kick into survival mode, and they will grow accustomed to not needing to eat all the time. These groundbreaking findings show that death from diabetes increased for children when the grandfather had a surplus of food and remarkably decreased when surplus food was available to the father.

This shows that nutrition can cause changes to genes that are passed down through generations in the male line and can affect the risk of developing diseases such as heart disease and diabetes. It is worth noting how health outcomes related to diabetes for subsequent generations are shaped based on one's grandfather's access to food during the slow growth period. Heart disease, on the other hand, was associated with the eating experiences of one's father, not grandfather.

Another study was done with mice that showed how diet during early development can have long-lasting effects on future generations.

Agouti mice have agouti genes that cause them to eat constantly, leading them to a life of obesity. This gene gives them yellow fur color and predisposes them to an early death of heart disease, cancer, and diabetes. Because they have the obese-yellow syndrome, even when food is restricted, these mice will become fatter on any amount of food they are given due to their gene.

In this experiment, researchers fed pregnant mice a methyl-rich diet of greens filled with folic acid, zinc, and B vitamins and then waited for the babies to be born. This study led to the birth of epigenetics.

By eating a diet full of greens, the obese-yellow mother was able to give birth to pups that were brown, lean, and stayed healthy for life. Although all mice with the agouti gene were genetically destined for a life of sickness, some were able to "turn their lives around" just by having their diets changed.

Generally speaking, mice and humans have shown to share virtually the same sets of genes.

These findings show that the environment in the mother's womb influences adult health, which is not only affected by what we eat but what our parents ate.

This also shows that what you do in life dictates your destiny—everything from your thoughts to the food you eat to your lifestyle habits.

The great news here is that you can influence your gene expression, and you can do it at any age. It's never too late to improve your health.

For instance, if you were born with one of the most lethal forms of the obesity gene, the FTO gene, you can take action now that will dampen the effect of the FTO gene, thereby preventing it from expressing. Such actions may include walking thirty minutes every day, losing weight, filling your body with phytonutrients and antioxidants, and eating healthy meals, including fruits and vegetables, whole grains, healthy fats, and beans.

Parents need to consider changing their eating and lifestyle habits decades before thinking of conceiving.

One study shows that young men who smoke before puberty (younger than eleven years old) give birth to sons who are more likely to become overweight in their teenage years. The study shows that overeating or exposure to toxins by the father at this key developmental stage leaves memory on sperm cells.

If you are born with an addictive gene for smoking, you can choose to do something about it. You can dampen it and mute it by taking steps to reduce nicotine exposure. Every try counts. Quitting smoking is possible. You can start by taking small steps. You can talk to your doctor or pharmacist who can assist you with nicotine replacement therapy to double your chances of quitting for good. Examples include nicotine gums, patches, and lozenges. Medication can also help, such as bupropion SR. You can identify triggers and learn strategies to manage your cravings by keeping busy. When a craving hits, choose to go for a walk instead. Choose to breathe through your craving and chew a sugarless gum. Don't have "just one," no matter how hard the urge.

You can change your negative thoughts with a positive mindset. You can say out loud, "I am enough. I am healed. I am healthy." You can change your gene expression with every single thought, every movement, and every diet choice. You can take control of your genetic destiny through positive thoughts, healthy lifestyle habits, and daily actions.

There was another experiment done on rats to investigate exposure to the herbicide glyphosate to see whether glyphosate can cause transgenerational effects. The findings showed that when the male great-grandchild of the exposed mother reached middle age, they developed the prostate disease. They also showed an increased risk for obesity in both themselves and their offspring.

Scientists are finding that air pollution can increase the risk of neurodegenerative diseases, such as Alzheimer's and Parkinson's. B vitamins may protect against the harmful epigenetic effects of pollution and their effect on the body.

Even at low doses and longer exposure, what impact could this have on our health and future generations?

Start combating your risk by supporting your immune system. Choose to take your vitamins.

Researchers have shown stories of identical twins who were separated at birth and grew up in different environments. Because identical twins develop from a single fertilized egg, any differences between them are from the environment rather than genetics.

In one case, one twin developed a disease early in life, and the other twin was not affected.

Studies show that, in fraternal twins, when one has schizophrenia, the other has a 10 to 15 percent chance of developing it as well, and identical twins have a 50 percent chance. Since identical twins share identical genetic makeup, why isn't that figure 100 percent? The fact that both identical twins do not develop the same disease 100 percent of the time simply means that other environmental factors are contributing to this. This shows that DNA alone is not enough to determine susceptibility to disease.

Identical twins are different even though they have the same genetic makeup. Recent studies have shown how large epigenetic differences are seen in genetically identical twins and the role they play.

In one study, one twin had autism spectrum disorder while the other twin was unaffected. In the twin with autism, the DNA methylation was different than in the unaffected twin. DNA methylation occurs when a methyl group is added to DNA to modify the function of the genes and how they're expressed, especially during early development. This data shows the important role that epigenetics plays in autism spectrum disorder. It would be interesting to see how these patterns affect their brain function.

Yet another study showed that when a woman lacks folate during pregnancy, there's a detrimental effect that persists to multiple generations. The researchers looked at a gene called methylenetetrahydrofolate reductase (MTHFR). The MTHFR gene is critical for breaking down one form of B vitamin, folate, into another. It's also part of the process for DNA repair and building new DNA in growing cells.

MTHFR abnormalities found in the maternal grandfather or maternal grandmother affected their grandchildren. Observed defects in the grandchildren included growth restriction, developmental delay, and neural tube defects. The study showed that these defects were not caused by genetic effects but rather an epigenetic effect. The MTHFR mutation is a change in DNA sequencing, caused by mistakes when DNA is copied. These replication errors are thought to be influenced by environmental factors, such as cigarette smoking, and can disrupt the genetic regulation in later generations.

Folate metabolism plays an epigenetic role during development, and these effects persist for multiple generations in the mouse model.

If you are predisposed to these kinds of disorders, how do you find the methyl to reprogram your genes? Eat your veggies. Have more positive thoughts. Increase your daily movement. If you're constantly craving sugar, salt, fast foods, fried chicken, and red meat, resist the urge and choose kale and whole foods instead. Just remember, you have the innate ability in you to change your very epigenome. You are your own destiny and can influence the strengthening of future generations as well.

What we do and what our environment is like affect gene expression. In other words, we are what our grandmother ate. The nutrition a mother gives a baby when she is pregnant not only comes from the food she eats but also from the body she made as a child.

The egg that made you was nourished by your grandmother. Epigenetic effects are passed down from one generation to the next.

Some studies on human populations are attempting to link human health effects to a cause. In one of these studies, evidence was found that prenatal and early postnatal environmental factors influence the risk of a child developing various chronic diseases in adulthood, such as obesity, cancer, and diabetes, and mental health issues such as behavioral disorders. These studies are pointing to the fact that environmental exposure early in development has a role in susceptibility to disease later in life.

Researchers confirm that very few genetic abnormalities are associated with disease. This means that very few diseases are genetic-based and that it is more common that the environment has a significant impact in causing the disease. Environmental factors like toxins and chemicals can induce disease by changing the epigenetics of the individual to cause adult-onset disease, which is then transferred to subsequent generations.

A change in the sperm or egg can permanently be programmed to not only occur in that person but in generations to come. It may be that we are seeing an increase in the number of people in a state of disease based on this continual increase in transgenerational epigenetics. What are you willing to do to protect not just your children from health issues but your grandchildren as well?

chapter 4

Are Epigenetic Changes Reversible?

Did you know that 90 percent of US men and 80 percent of women have excess belly fat? This is no joke because excess belly fat, also known as visceral fat, poses serious health risks. Regardless of your overall weight, carrying extra weight around your belly is linked to preventable health issues such as high blood pressure, sleep apnea, gout, osteoarthritis, insulin resistance, and type 2 diabetes. It can even increase the risk of premature death.

It is important to know your waist measurement so that you can choose to take the necessary steps to fix the problem. To check if you have too much belly fat, place a measuring tape right above your hipbone and measure your waist. For men, if your waist is more than forty inches around, you have unhealthy fat. This poses a greater risk of health problems. The same health risks apply to women with waists over thirty-five inches around.

As a clinical pharmacist, I help patients prevent harmful side effects of their medication and make sure their medications are safe, effective, and affordable. I focus on disease prevention through optimizing my patients' health with the right medications, alternative therapies, nutritional supplements, self-care, and lifestyle interventions. I offer medication therapy management (MTM) services and health coaching where I sit one on one with patients, or offer virtual consultations to check for any medication-related problems, to educate my patients and collaborate with their health care providers for an optimal health outcome.

In one of these sessions, I met David, a fifty-two-year-old man with multiple chronic conditions taking multiple medications. He was on medications for high blood pressure, type 2 diabetes, and high cholesterol, none of which were well controlled.

I listened actively as David told me he had started getting chest pains six months prior and had been ignoring the symptoms. Instead of getting the chest pain checked out, he would go to the pharmacy instead and get a bottle of Tums. It's important to learn how to listen to your body and to get to know what your body wants.

One morning, David woke up to the worst chest pain of all time. The pain started in his chest and radiated to his neck, making breathing very painful for him. He went to the emergency room, where he was diagnosed with a silent heart attack. He couldn't believe it. He was a family man, active and full of life. However, he was also working double shifts, eating whatever he wanted, and had no time to sleep at night. Sometimes, if we don't take the time to listen to what our body is saying, it may force us to slow down, whether we like it or not.

He was immediately scheduled for open-heart surgery to remove the blockage in his artery. He had a cardiac catheterization done and a stent placed in his heart. For a few months, he slowed down his fast-paced life, and he was doing well with healing from his procedure. But this only worked for a short time. Before he knew it, he started getting chest pain again, leading him in and out of the hospital. He shared with me that he's had thirty cardiac catheterizations and over ten stents put in. And he's only fifty-two!

After listening to his story, I started asking him more open-ended questions so that together we could get to the root cause of the problem.

I asked him about his eating habits since we now know that half of all deaths due to type 2 diabetes, stroke, and heart disease start with poor food choices.

He said he regularly ate foods such as fried eggs, smoked bacon, sausages, red meat, white bread, white rice, pizza, French fries, fried chicken, potato chips, and ice cream, and he drank soda and alcohol regularly.

I asked him what would motivate him to make positive changes to his health and, with regard to the massive number of stents and medical procedures he'd had, to fix his poor health choices. I asked him at what point would enough be enough.

He expressed frustration because he had thought the heart surgery would take care of all his chest pain problems. He couldn't understand why he had to keep coming back for new stents, why he was getting sicker and sicker, and why new medications kept being added to his regimen.

He told me that he was a father of three teenage boys, the husband of a beautiful wife, an active member in his community, and a jolly fellow. He told me he was worried sick about his family, especially about what might happen to them in his absence. He talked about his desire to watch his children grow up and his goals in life.

I empathized with David about his past miseries and encouraged him to understand that he has the freedom to choose to live better through lifestyle changes and to stay out of the hospital and live a longer, healthier life.

I pointed out to him that he had two choices to make that day: he could either make a drastic change to his dietary choices and change his body's trajectory or choose to continue his old lifestyle habits and keep getting the same results.

You know your body better than any doctor ever will. Isn't it time to start listening to what your body is saying and to start making better choices? Your health is in your own hands; stop outsourcing it to others.

Thirty percent of health care spending is wasted on procedures that could be prevented. The cost of health care is going through the roof at an unsustainable rate.

With all the stents in David's heart, all the trips to the ER, the chest pains, and all the medications he was taking on a daily basis, unfortunately his health was already far gone, and he was not showing signs of getting better.

It broke my heart to see him go through all these health issues that were potentially preventable. It is overwhelming to think about the number of people who have this same problem.

Isn't it time to get to the root cause of the problem? Most diseases don't start overnight, and most chronic conditions don't happen randomly. Genetically susceptible people, which is most of us, make lifestyle choices and take daily actions that lead to consequences that affect our health outcomes for generations to come.

Your genes can contribute to your chances of being overweight or obese, but balancing the calories you consume with movement, strength training exercises, a healthy diet, reduced portion size, and replacing sugary beverages with adequate water intake can prevent weight gain and dampen this obese gene from expressing.

New studies suggest that certain foods and supplements may be able to alter our gene expression and improve or worsen our health outcomes.

We can choose fresh, whole foods and let go of bagged, boxed, or packaged foods. We have the choice to replace alcohol and sodas with water and to switch animal proteins such as red meat and bacon to plant-based protein such as beans, nuts, and legumes. We have the option to eat five to thirteen cups of fresh fruits and vegetables a day and to opt for whole grains, such as brown rice and quinoa, instead of white bread or white pasta. We have to make the choices to reduce sugar, oil, and salt in our food choices or snacks and to choose organic and natural foods and household items to lessen our environmental exposures to toxins. We even have the choice to become physically active by moving our bodies more. Examples include taking thirty-minute daily walks and strength training weekly with exercises such as eight reps of push-ups, sit-ups, chin-ups, squat thrusts, lunges, weight lifting, and step-ups. You can choose to lose weight and spend more time outdoors. These are all steps toward reversing bad epigenetic changes to reduce disease risks and improve health outcomes.

Your mother's or father's experiences as a child and their lifestyle choices as adults may have shaped your epigenome, but they can be reversed.

Our genes are composed of variations of protein bases. While there are only four possible bases (adenine, thymine, guanine, and cytosine), they can be grouped together in various combinations to code for countless functions in the body. These four bases make up the DNA sequence and combine to form instructions that tell your body how to function properly.

Sometimes, when cells in the body duplicate to make new cells, mistakes are made. A mistake in just one letter can alter the meaning or function of a gene. These variations are called single nucleotide polymorphisms, or SNPs.

These small variations in DNA are expressed in multiple ways. They can influence how we break down food and what types of exercises are best for our bodies. By determining our own unique gene variations, we can tailor lifestyle approaches and nutritional supplementation to boost our genetic potential to improve our health outcomes to live longer, healthier lives.

I have done hundreds of consultations with patients on personalized services like gene SNP analysis testing. With gene SNP analysis, you can gain valuable information about your gene expression and its impact on factors that may contribute to chronic health concerns. It looks into what roles your genes play in your digestive health, how well your body copes with the stress of physical activity, and how environmental factors affect your body and, in doing so, helps you find accurately tailored answers for what a healthy lifestyle looks like to you.

Dietary intervention based on knowledge of nutritional status and genetic makeup can be used to prevent, reduce, or combat chronic disease.

The solution to finding the root cause is in our daily lifestyle choices and habits. You have the power inside of you to choose to live a better lifestyle. Your body has the innate ability to heal itself, given a chance. Now that you have this information, what are you going to do with it?

chapter five

Your Health Matters

Have you ever paused to think about the chemicals you're exposed to daily? Are you worried about your family's exposure to toxic chemicals in and outside the home? How can you promote healthy living at home?

Pesticides are chemicals used to protect crops from insects, weeds, and infections that often tamper with the crops' growth and development. Unfortunately, we get exposed to these toxins by eating them in our food. Pesticides are sprayed on fruits, vegetables, wheat, rice, and more. Pesticides are even fed to the very animals whose meat we buy and eat regularly. Even unborn babies are exposed to them through their mother's diet and infants through breast milk. No one has a free pass; we are all exposed!

Over 13 million deaths worldwide are associated with environmental pollutants. These environmental toxins are responsible for 24 percent of potentially preventable diseases every year. If you think ingesting them is harmless, think again.

The CDC performed daily exposure screening tests, and the results were stunning. There were 148 different environmental chemicals found in the blood and urine of the US population.

Many household cleaning products on the market are extremely toxic. Just because these products made it to the store shelves doesn't guarantee their safety. The manufacturers of these products are not required to disclose even the active ingredients in products such as laundry detergents, glass cleaners, dish soap, wipes, and more.

The World Health Organization (WHO) estimates 30–40 percent of the burden of childhood disease is due to environmental factors. There are 80,000–150,000 registered chemicals for which we have no known information, meaning they're not regulated. We use hundreds of these chemicals daily and have continuous exposure to these toxins through eating them in our food, using them as the cream we rub on our skin and makeup we put on our faces, washing the clothes we wear, using soap to wash ourselves, and even just breathing them in through the air. These toxins are constantly around us, which contributes to many inflammatory processes that lead to many diseases. Growing evidence suggests that environmental pollutants may cause diseases through epigenetic gene expression changes.

Heavy metals, especially, are environmental toxins associated with various diseases.

Arsenic has been linked to various cancers and schizophrenia. Nickel has been linked to heart disease, various cancers, and diabetic nephropathy. And cadmium has been linked to colorectal cancer, kidney cancers, and cancers of the blood and bone marrow.

A developing baby given bisphenol A (BPA), an endocrine disruptor with a reproductive effect, may be linked to increased cancer risk in adult life. BPA can leach into food through plastic containers, baby bottles, and tooth-colored dental filling materials. BPA can also cause epigenetic abnormalities with prenatal exposure, leading to the deterioration of brain functions such as memory and cognition even after the children have grown.

So how is this important? What does this mean for our exposure to plastics? Could they have something to do with all the health issues we have today? You can start by not reheating your food in the microwave in plastic containers, except those labeled as microwave safe. You can choose to use glass and ceramic containers that do not contain a metal rim to reheat your food. You can also choose the oven, convection toaster oven, air fryers, steamers, or stovetops as microwave alternative.

Our fruits and vegetables are also sprayed with pesticides. Some are treated with ripening and coating agents, and some are sprayed with white powders to preserve the moisture and prevent sogginess, so they remain fresh when they get to the grocery stores.

Research shows that washing our fruits and vegetables with running water alone does not remove these chemical residues.

A safer alternative is to buy organic foods that contain fewer chemicals. Unfortunately, most people cannot afford to go all organic. So how do we stay safe and reduce our exposure to toxins from the food we consume?

Make the choice to buy local produce in season or grow your own produce. Try as much as possible to only buy unpackaged fruits and vegetables and avoid packaged and processed foods.

Every time you buy your produce, get in the habit of soaking your fruits and vegetables in water and add one tablespoon of baking soda (sodium bicarbonate is an alkalizing agent) into the container. Leave them to soak for fifteen to twenty minutes and wash them thoroughly with warm water. A better alternative option is to invest in a smart food cleaner to instantly eliminate pesticides and insecticides from conventional as well as organic produce.

Get to know which fruits and vegetables have higher levels of pesticide residue and choose wisely.

Choose to make the majority of your diet plant-based. Leafy green vegetables have high-alkaline properties. The alkaline minerals in our bodies are used to neutralize acidic conditions caused by the environment, and since green vegetables help replenish our alkaline mineral stores, they help us filter out pollutants.

Choose to limit animal-based products such as red meat, high-mercury fish, fried chicken, pork, and canned meat products. Limit animal products, including dairy products, to twice a month or less and consume them in smaller portion sizes.

Choose to avoid eating "unclean" animals—in other words, animals whose meat is toxic and makes us sick. Flesh food is inferior to a plant-based diet, and eating toxic foods limits our usefulness for God. The Bible says: "Ye shall not make yourselves abominable with any creeping thing that creepeth, neither shall ye make yourselves unclean with them, that ye should be defiled thereby. For I am the Lord your God: Ye shall therefore sanctify yourselves, and ye shall be holy; for I am holy: neither shall ye defile yourselves with any manner of creeping thing that creepeth upon the earth" (Leviticus 11:43–44, KJV).

Examples of unclean animals are pigs, crabs, owls, badgers, rabbits, kites, electric eels, falcons, chameleons, hoopoes, seagulls, eagles, herons, and lizards.

Choose to avoid ingredients such as artificial sweeteners, refined sugar, monosodium glutamate (MSG), artificial colors, butylated hydroxytoluene

(BHT), sodium nitrate, olestra, brominated vegetable oil, pesticides, and genetically modified organisms (GMOs) when cooking.

The Environmental Working Group identifies the types of produce most likely to be contaminated with pesticides as apples, celery, sweet bell peppers, peaches, strawberries, grapes, spinach, green beans, kale, lettuce, cucumbers, blueberries, and potatoes. They recommend eating organic versions of these "dirty dozen" fruits and vegetables. We can eat more of onions, sweet corn, pineapple, avocado, cabbage, sweet peas, asparagus, mangoes, eggplant, kiwi, cantaloupe, sweet potatoes, grapefruit, watermelon, and mushrooms. They have thick outer skins that prevent pesticides from touching the edible inside, making them safer to eat. We should eat a wide variety of fruits and vegetables every day with our meals to get the most health benefits and protection against disease.

Since most fruits and vegetables in the supermarket are full of chemicals, choose organic when you can but know that organic produce can be expensive. Patients ask me all the time how to supplement their diet while avoiding paying the high price of organic fruits and vegetables. Supper Greens are a unique variety of superfood. An example is an affordable, yet powerful product called Complete Greens to those whose daily routine is lacking in nutrients. It is organic and comes in isotonic formulation to give rapid absorption of the powerful nutrients you need. The formula features a combination of natural ingredients like alfalfa grass, wheatgrass, and chlorella, which help you make your body more alkaline to reduce inflammation. It also contains extract from whole foods like broccoli powder, cabbage powder, and spinach powder, which help detoxify your body.

To better protect your health, stick with USDA Certified Organic label, with lower detectable levels of pesticide residue. I encourage you to do your own research and become well informed, so you can make wise decisions about what to put into your body.

chapter six

The Power of Nutrition in Transforming Health

Around the year 1900, Native Americans and Alaska Natives lived by hunting, fishing, gathering, and farming. But as times changed, so did their way of life.

Common chronic diseases that are rampant today, such as obesity, type 2 diabetes, heart disease, and cancer, were once very rare. These people ate traditional plant-rich, high-fiber diets and were always on the move. Everyone ate different varieties and colors of vegetables every day.

The children in the communities gathered and played traditional games, as well as soccer, football, and basketball; they were always playing outdoors.

After 1950, their way of life changed drastically. They started adopting a more "Western" diet. They started eating more processed foods, such as microwave popcorn, instant ramen, frozen dinners, and processed meats like bacon and hot dogs. They ate more foods high in sugar and industrial fats like French fries, donuts, frozen pizza, and foods low in fiber. They were hardly eating any vegetables at all.

There was once a time when people ate fresh fruit in its whole form, but now they drink fruits as juices filled with loads of corn syrups and artificial sweeteners. Nowadays, there is an increase in disease with skyrocketing rates of diabetes, obesity, and cancer.

Likewise, children in the community are staying indoors more often and playing video games all day such as Playstation 5 and Xbox Series. Social media has taken over the socialization with peers that children used to get from more traditional games and sports. With a lack of physical activity and the indulgence in more processed foods, children and adults alike are becoming more overweight. In native nations, young people are now at greater risk for type 2 diabetes.

This problem extends to African nations as well. For instance, West Africa has an ongoing problem in addressing undernutrition. However, as the population moved from rural areas to more urban ones, they started to experience more technological development, and their dietary patterns and physical activity levels changed. The childhood and adult obesity rate skyrocketed.

There was once a time when everybody cooked at home and ate healthily, but if you travel to African countries today, you will see fast-food franchises like KFC and McDonalds. Native people are becoming attracted to eating more fast foods because they believe Western foods are superior and taste better. Because of this, they are suffering from many modern chronic diseases as well.

We are seeing a lower consumption of fruits and vegetables universally in West Africa even though there is mass production of this kind of product in the land. The adult obesity rate has increased by 115 percent since 2004 in West Africa.

A history of poor eating habits and the lack of physical activity have contributed significantly to the health-related issues that many face today in the US. More than two-thirds of adults and nearly one-third of children are overweight or obese.

What we eat matters. More specifically, the quality of the food we eat matters.

The food you eat enters your bloodstream and creates your cells, tissues, and organs. Therefore, the quality of the food you eat is essential. Not only does it affect your cells, but it also affects your mood, your skin quality, your hair, your immune system, and everything else.

Recent studies indicate that the food you eat can change your genes and potentially change the genes of your children and even future generations. How?

Let's consider the importance of good nutrition during pregnancy. Women need to take adequate folic acid (400 mcg of folic acid daily) supplementation way before they get pregnant and especially during early pregnancy, the first trimester (800 mcg to 1 mg folic acid daily), because it can prevent serious medical problems, such as neural tube defects in the brain and spine of the baby.

One study showed what happened in the western Netherlands in the winter between 1944 and 1945. There was a terrible famine that forced everybody, including those pregnant at the time, to go on a calorie-restricted diet of fewer than one thousand calories per day. Normally, you are supposed to eat for two during pregnancy, but, unfortunately, these pregnant women had to go to bed hungry many nights, eating just between four hundred and eight hundred calories a day. A group of scientists followed these pregnant women over time to observe what would happen when they delivered their babies down the road. Interestingly, they found elevated rates of obesity and heart problems in the children, now full-grown adults sixty years later, compared to their siblings who were not born during this famine period. What happens during those first few months of pregnancy, during which the baby is developing, is crucial, and it determines much about their future health.

The people exposed to famine in their mother's womb had a low degree of methylation (addition of a methyl group) of a gene involved in insulin breakdown (the insulin-like growth factor 2 gene). Looking at this from another angle, this means that changing your diet before conceiving could potentially help stop poor health outcomes later in life.

What you eat, especially during the early developmental period, may have a profound impact on disease for the child later in life, and the effect may carry on to future generations as well.

It is important to know that malnutrition in early life can correlate to chronic conditions in adulthood.

A Western diet that included fried chicken, refined grains, prepackaged foods, and sweetened beverages was found in another study to reduce the production of important chemicals such as short-chain fatty acids (SCFAs). SCFAs, like butyrate, are fatty acids produced by gut bacteria in the large intestine to support immune function and to supply energy to the cells of the gut. Good gut bacteria ferment and break down nondigestible fibers like fruits and vegetables to produce SCFAs. Foods high in fiber allow good gut bacteria to thrive and provide epigenetic protection against disease development. However, eating processed foods and drinking sugary drinks can shift the ratio of the good and bad gut bacteria, which significantly reduces the production of these important SCFAs, leading to alterations in gene expression and subsequently gut-related diseases, such as Crohn's disease, ulcerative colitis, irritable bowel syndrome, and colorectal cancer.

Your diet can change your sperm DNA and can also be passed on to future generations. In one study, researchers fed male mice a poor diet, causing the mice to become obese and later develop type 2 diabetes. When those male mice had female offspring, the offspring were fed a normal diet and grew up with a healthy weight. Even so, the offspring developed type 1 diabetes. Why is that? It turns out that the high inflammatory diet fed to the male mice caused epigenetic marks that caused methyl groups to attach to the sperm DNA next to the gene important for creating insulin in the pancreas and turned them off one by one. It rendered them useless, in other words, the DNA was not able to make any insulin, leading to a greater risk of developing type 1 diabetes.

In another study done on humans, sperm DNA samples were taken from obese men and were compared to those of lean men. They found the sperm DNA from the obese men had many epigenetic marks (methyl groups) in many different places not seen on those of the lean men. Later, the obese men underwent bariatric surgery, which caused a lot of their excess weight to come off. Their sperm DNA was collected a week after and then a year after. Fascinatingly, in that one week, the epigenetic marks on the sperm DNA had changed drastically, and in one year, it looked just like those of lean men. Just weight loss alone was able to change sperm DNA. This shows that lifestyle changes like losing weight and improving your diet choices work!

The nutrients in different foods may reverse epigenetic patterns.

Our genes influence the way we absorb and metabolize micronutrients and can also influence which genes are turned on or off.

Micronutrients are needed in our body to assist in performing certain necessary reactions the enzymes cannot perform alone. Unfortunately, many people have certain genetic polymorphisms that prevent them from activating these genes. Dr. Rhonda Patrick is a biomedical science researcher on micronutrient deficiencies and how genetics affects how the body processes nutrition. She mentioned in her research that people respond differently to different types of diets and to different macronutrients as well as micronutrients.

Some examples of macronutrients are fat, protein, dietary fiber, and carbohydrates. These are needed in a large amount in our diet. Micronutrients include vitamins and minerals needed in a small amount but are vital to development, disease prevention, and our total well-being. Since micronutrients are not produced in the body, they must be derived from our diet.

For instance, magnesium is needed for more than three hundred biochemical reactions in the body. It helps to maintain normal nerve and muscle function, supports a healthy immune system, keeps the heartbeat steady, helps adjust blood glucose, helps in the production of energy and protein, and helps bones remain strong. The TRPM6 gene polymorphism carries magnesium from the food we eat, such as seeds, nuts, kale, and spinach, into our cells. If you happen to have this TRPM6 polymorphism, you have a two-fold higher risk for type 2 diabetes when your magnesium level is low (the normal level is between 250 mg and 400 mg/day). Forty-five percent of people have inadequate magnesium levels. Ask your doctor to check your magnesium levels if you experience the following symptoms: muscle cramps or twitches, fatigue or muscle weakness, irregular heartbeat, constipation, or nausea and vomiting.

Vitamin D deficiency is also very common. It's estimated that about one billion people worldwide have low levels of this vitamin in their blood. Vitamin D is a steroid hormone and regulates over one thousand genes in the body. When we get vitamin D from the sun through UVB radiation, it hits our skin and gets converted to something in our gene called 7-dehydrocholesterol, which then converts into vitamin D_3. Older people cannot do this very well as their skin thins with age and vitamin D synthesis becomes less efficient. Some people have a problem converting vitamin D_3 into the active form of vitamin D and need optimal levels than people without that gene variation. People with darker skin also have a problem because the melanin in dark skin doesn't absorb as much UV radiation. So the darker your skin color, the less likely you are to absorb vitamin D from the sun and the more at risk of being deficient you are. Where you live can also affect vitamin D absorption. Your use of sunscreen can also affect it, as can the health of your gut. Conditions that affect the gut and digestion, such as celiac disease, chronic pancreatitis, Crohn's disease, and cystic fibrosis, can reduce vitamin D absorption. You may very well be getting good exposure to the sun but not absorbing the benefit. Being overweight or obese may also put you at risk for vitamin D deficiency, as will staying indoors most of the day. If you get sick often, always feel tired, have bone pain in your legs, or are feeling depressed, talk to your doctor about ordering a test called 25-hydroxy vitamin D blood test to see if a vitamin D_3 supplement might benefit you.

Another example is a gene polymorphism called peroxisome proliferator-activated receptor (PPAR gamma), which is needed to metabolize fatty acids. If people with this gene have low levels of good fat and high intake of bad fats, such as red meat and dairy products, they have a much higher risk of developing obesity and type 2 diabetes.

When you fry meat at very high temperatures regularly, the meat can form a dangerous chemical called heterocyclic amine, which can eventually become a carcinogen and cause cancer. Fortunately, humans have a gene called NAT2, which can inactivate heterocyclic amine. However, many people have slow NAT2 activity, and eating bad fats and processed foods regularly may make the process so slow that some heterocyclic amine isn't deactivated, which may dramatically increase the risk of cancer.

It's up to each of us to take care of ourselves. Know your genes and how to change the expression of your genes in your lifetime. Know what your body wants. But how do you know what genes you have and what you are predisposed to? This is where personalized medicine and gene SNP analysis comes in. I have done hundreds of these personalized nutritional health reports and have interpreted the results for what dietary and lifestyle solutions may help to better deal with any predispositions to a disease they may have. Consider getting this personalized test done so you won't have to guess anymore.

Blueberries are high in antioxidants and may epigenetically reduce DNA damage, slow the aging process, and protect us from getting cancer.

Tomatoes contain lycopene, a powerful antioxidant, which combats free radicals that are harmful to our bodies. They are good for our blood and heart.

Cruciferous vegetables (bok choy, broccoli, Brussels sprouts, cabbage, and cauliflower) activate genes that can prevent cancer development through a compound called sulforaphane.

Foods high in omega-3 fatty acids can decrease inflammation and protect tissues from inflammatory damage. For most people, an omega-6 to omega-3 ratio of 4:1 is recommended, meaning four omega-6s for every omega-3. Antiaging experts suggest maintaining a 1:1 ratio in favor of omega-3s. However, most Americans eat a ratio of anywhere from 20:1 to 25:1 omega-6 to omega-3. This is very bad as it raises the risk of all sorts of serious modern lifestyle diseases, such as type 2 diabetes, cancer, and heart disease.

Examples of good fats are avocado, cold-pressed olive oil, walnuts, flaxseed, and fish fats or high-quality omega-3 fatty acid supplements. Avoid vegetable oils loaded with omega-6 fatty acids, such as soybean oil, sunflower oil, corn oil, and cottonseed oil.

Keep in mind that limiting the amount of animal and processed foods in your diet can help reduce inflammation.

Dark leafy greens are essential for reducing inflammation. Beta-carotene, vitamin C, and flavonoids like quercetin are powerful anti-inflammatory agents found in vegetables.

Green vegetables are the most commonly missing food in modern diets. Learning to add dark leafy greens to your diet is essential to establishing a healthy body and immune system. When you nourish yourself with greens, you are eliminating foods that make you sick.

If you get bored with your favorite vegetables, be adventurous and try kinds that you've never tried before.

Remember, some greens like spinach, Swiss chard, and beet greens should be eaten in moderation because they are high in oxalic acid, which may block the absorption of the calcium these foods contain.

Choose quality whole grains. Brown rice, kasha, millet, and quinoa are all examples of great grains. Each of these whole grains contains fiber, B vitamins, minerals, and protein. Whole grains support balanced blood sugar levels and digestion and help you feel satisfied. This means you can stay fuller longer and avoid the urge to overeat, thus supporting a healthy weight.

Your epigenetic patterns change based on what you eat, how much you sleep, how you exercise, and what substances you are exposed to. All these changes can ultimately influence your risk of developing chronic conditions such as heart disease or type 2 diabetes.

What you choose to eat, starting from one meal, extending to what you eat through the year, and in your lifetime can alter your epigenetics, your behavior, and everything about you.

You have the power to make choices to avoid industrial foods and go back to the basics for your health. An ancestral diet includes eating wholesome, natural, and organic foods, prepared by using indigenous ingredients that sustained our ancestors for many, many years.

Family history may be a strong predictor of disease, but we have the power to change it. This means that we are not completely at the mercy of our genes. The truth is our genes are at the mercy of our food choices, lifestyle decisions, and daily habits. Therefore, choose to eat healthy foods. Choose to stay active. Make wise choices. Join the healthy lifestyle movement today and do it for you, your children, and future generations.

chapter seven

Gut Health Issues Linked With Epigenetic Changes

Gut health is the key to good health. Evidence shows that many chronic metabolic conditions are influenced by chronic gut inflammation. Gut health is connected to everything that happens in our body, and therefore it is also directly linked to the formation of disease. If your gut isn't functioning well, other organ systems will not function optimally either.

Bloating, stomach pain, constipation, adrenal fatigue, skin disorders, acne, insomnia, and mental and emotional states are all connected to the gut. It is estimated that at least 60 million Americans are affected by a digestive disease. This is becoming an epidemic. There is an old saying, "Death begins in the colon."

Some digestive diseases are gastrointestinal reflux disease (GERD)/heartburn, irritable bowel syndrome (IBS), constipation, diarrhea, gallstones, liver disease, celiac disease, gluten-related disorders, diverticulitis disease, and inflammatory bowel disease, such as Crohn's or ulcerative colitis.

How do you turn off genes to prevent future disease? One study found that eating well can "turn off" the heart attack genes that put one at higher risk for heart problems. In this study, people who ate more raw fruits and vegetables had a reduced risk of heart disease, even if they carried copies of the gene that increases the risk for cardiovascular disease. It's all about the gut.

So how can you improve your gut health? It's important to understand microbes. Microbes are tiny living things found everywhere around us and are too small to see with our naked eyes. They are beneficial to life, but some kinds can also cause serious harm. Millions of these microorganisms live in our digestive tract, where they regulate and balance the gut. Any major shift in their composition can lead to disorders such as inflammatory bowel disease, allergies, autoimmune disease, diabetes, mental disorders, and cancer.

A microbiome is a diverse community of various microorganisms with their sets of genes that reside in us. They include bacteria, fungi, algae, protozoa, viruses, and parasites. Their inhabitants are diverse, and microbiomes vary from one person to another. These different bacteria species reside in the mouth, skin, gut, vagina, and so on. The microbiome varies greatly among different body sites, and they change over time in response to factors such as the food we eat, our genetics, and the environment we live in.

There are good and bad bacteria. Out of the total bacteria in our bodies, to stay healthy we need a ratio of about 85 percent good bacteria to 15 percent bad bacteria, so our immune system is strong but still on alert to protect us. Whenever there is an imbalance in this ratio, we have something called dysbiosis, an imbalance in the microbial community. Imbalances can cause disease. There are strong correlations between the human gut microbiome and conditions such as obesity, type 2 diabetes, and inflammatory bowel disease.

To get to the root cause of your gut health issues, you should consider answering these questions:

- How healthy are/were your mother and father? Do they suffer from many kinds of chronic diseases? Do they take multiple medications? Have they undergone multiple surgeries? Are they still alive?
- What kind of childhood diseases did you have?
- Did you take antibiotics regularly growing up?
- Were you birthed normally or through Cesarean (C-section)?

Babies born via C-section may be at risk for developing future illnesses because the biome is never properly established. They did not get the initial good bacterial load at childbirth.

Babies born by caesarean section are exposed to different strains of bacteria as compared to babies born vaginally. New research shows babies born via c-section may have a weaker immune system, which may affect their health later in life because of a lack of exposure to their mother's bacteria. Epidemiological studies suggested that they have a greater risk of asthma and obesity later in life. While some mothers are requesting "vaginal seeding" to correct this issue, which is the process of transferring the mother's vaginal flora to babies born via c-section who haven't received that exposure, the American College of Obstetricians and Gynecologists has warned against the practice due to concerns over the potential risk of transferring pathogenic organisms from the mom to her baby.

- Were you breastfed or formula-fed? Another factor affecting the microbiome is breastfeeding. Breastfed infants are exposed to more beneficial bacteria from their mothers than formula-fed babies. It is highly encouraged that mothers breastfeed their children for at least one year because of the many, many benefits to both the mothers and their babies. Breastfeeding has been shown to protect babies from getting many infections as well as protection against serious health problems and hospitalization. Moreover, It's been shown to also protect mothers by lowering cancer risks. Researchers found more than seven hundred species of microbes in breast milk, including colostrum. The American Academy of Pediatrics recommends that children can supplement with other proper complementary food starting after 6 months of exclusive breastfeeding. The longer you continue to breastfeed your child, the better for the baby's optimal health. If you are not able to breastfeed exclusively for the long term, you can ask your pediatrician about using infant formulas that contain ingredients such as probiotics, prebiotics, and nondigestible fibers.

One study found that populations of bacteria in the gut are highly sensitive to the food you eat. You are what you eat, as are the bacteria that live inside of you. You can, therefore, work to create a healthier diversity of good bacteria by paying more attention to what you eat.

Diet has a profound impact on the types of bacteria that thrive. Even a brief dietary change has been shown to alter the gut microbiota.

Both your long-term diet habits as well as short-term changes can lead to shifts in the kinds of microbes you have.

Let's address the long-term impact of diet on the gut microbiota. The diet a person eats over a year is strongly correlated with the combination of the gut microbiota.

For instance, people who eat a lot of carbohydrates, such as pasta, white rice, and potatoes, tend to have a lot of one kind of microorganism, while people who eat lots of protein, especially meat, will have a lot of a different kind.

Plant-based diets are especially supportive of the beneficial organisms in the gut.

A study demonstrated that a more extreme diet change can lead to more extreme microbiota changes over a short time. In this study, volunteers changed their diet dramatically for three days. Some volunteers went vegan, and some ate a "meat-and-cheese-only" diet.

The vegan diet caused a little change, but the meat-and-cheese diet caused big changes almost overnight. In the meat-and-cheese group, there was an increase in bacteria linked to cardiovascular disease. The results showed that the Western diet, heavy in meat and cheese, can alter the genetic composition and metabolic activity of our microorganisms and is suspected of contributing to the growing epidemic of chronic diseases, such as obesity and inflammatory bowel disease.

To change your microbiota to have more beneficial bacteria, you may do well to consider eating more plant-based foods in their most natural state and avoiding animal proteins, added sugar, and processed foods. In other words, eat more whole, natural foods.

Antibiotics can also affect the microbiome. Data from a 2016 study suggests that exposure to antibiotics in infancy can alter the gut microbiome and weaken the immune response for years to come.

Antibiotics work by killing bacteria. This is effective when you're sick and need help ridding yourself of harmful bacteria. However, they also cause collateral damage to the good bacteria that live in your gut. Even one dose of a commonly prescribed antibiotic can wipe out microbial diversity for up to one month. Antibiotics may cut down the bacteria in your gut like a lawnmower cuts grass.

Sixty percent of our antibiotic use in the United States is unnecessary, which is why there is so much antibiotic resistance.

It has been shown that gut microbiota is not the same in every person, and as a result, the time it takes to recover to the original gut microbiota after antibiotic use is different from person to person.

For instance, after a sickness for which you've had to take antibiotics, your children may bounce back right away, while your husband may take a few days and you may take a few months based on how strong or weak your immune system is.

Antibiotics are necessary at times, but remember to take extra precaution by talking to your doctor or pharmacist about taking a probiotic supplement following such treatment. Take care of your gut bacteria and watch that ratio!

At about one year of age, our gut microbial communities are much more diverse than when we were born, and they continue to develop as we eat more solid foods.

Once we reach adulthood, our microbial communities become highly complex.

Microbial diversity sometimes decreases after age seventy-five. As we move into old age, we begin to lose some of the stability that we had as younger adults. The composition of our gut's microbial communities shifts, changing from day to day and week to week.

Even brief periods of stress have been shown to alter the gut microbiota. Over the short term, stress can cause stomach aches, nausea, and diarrhea. In the long term, prolonged stress can aggravate chronic diseases such as irritable bowel syndrome and heartburn.

Poor sleep is associated with upper and lower gastrointestinal symptoms. Even the lack of sleep over a short time can change how your gut works.

Remove trigger foods such as gluten, dairy, eggs, corn, and highly processed foods, as well as toxins and alcohol. This reduces gas, bloating, and stomach pain. Eliminate suspect foods for twenty-one days under the close supervision of your physician. Work with your health care providers to start reintroducing one food back every four days and monitor for responses such as bloating, tiredness, sleep issues, skin reactions, and unhealthy bowel movements.

Take high-quality digestive enzymes to optimize digestive function. Also, add supportive gut-healing foods and herbs into your diet to nourish your gut. Foods to add include leafy greens, fruits, vegetables, quality fats, and proteins. Eat whole foods as much as possible. Add herbs to your meals instead of just using salt and pepper! For instance, turmeric is known to reduce inflammation. Thyme and oregano have antibacterial properties. Always make sure to check with your health care providers before adding herbs to your diet because some herbs may dangerously interact with medications you are taking and may not be right for those with certain health conditions. Do not start any new herbs during pregnancy without first consulting your health care provider.

Populate your microbiome with probiotic microflora to regulate bowel movement and prevent overgrowth of yeast.

Certain foods, such as lower glycemic foods and foods high in omega-3 fatty acids and antioxidants, can decrease inflammation and protect tissues from inflammatory damage. Examples of good fats are olive oil, nuts, and avocados.

Both probiotics and prebiotics help support gut health in different ways. Probiotics are helpful live bacteria that, when ingested, enhance the health of your gut.

These beneficial bacteria can alter the gut microflora, which in turn can change the production of dietary metabolites and modulate epigenetic-related processes like that of gut microbes.

Prebiotics are fibers that ferment in the gut and cause reactions in the body that promote good health. Examples are artichokes, leeks, chicory root, onions, quinoa, and amaranth.

Optimizing a balanced digestive system helps support your body's defenses. Having the right nutritional supplements in your regimen can support gut health and promote a healthy gene environment.

Poor nutrition can cause dysbiosis, which can, in turn, cause epigenetic changes that result in the onset and progression of certain diseases.

The good news is that many of these gut health issues are reversible once the gut problems are fixed.

chapter eight

How To Choose the Right Nutritional Supplements

Keep in mind that these statements have not been evaluated by the Food and Drug Administration (FDA). These products are not intended to diagnose, treat, cure, or prevent any disease.

In previous chapters, we learned from animal studies that a methyl-deficient diet such as low folate can cause certain parts of a genome—the complete assembly of your DNA that makes you unique—to be undermethylated for life and even affect future generations.

We also learned that your mother's diet during pregnancy and your diet in the early years can influence your epigenome and follow you into adulthood. To reiterate, the epigenome is a multitude of chemical compounds that tell the genome what to do.

As we better understand the connection between our diet and our epigenome, we can see why learning our own methylation patterns is crucial to improving our health outcomes.

The good news is that the changes caused by poor diet are reversible when methyl is added back into the diet.

Air pollution is also a major public health concern. A study showed that taking B vitamins can be used to reduce the impact of air pollution on the epigenome.

Another study showed that cancer is a preventable disease that requires major lifestyle changes.

Emerging studies reveal that only 5–10 percent of cancer incidences are exclusively caused by genetic factors. In most other cases, epigenetic alterations play an important part. The remaining 90–95 percent have their roots in environmental factors and lifestyle habits. They include cigarette smoking, poor diet choices, alcohol consumption, exposure to carcinogens in the air and water, infections, stress, obesity, and physical inactivity. As many as 30–35 percent of cancer cases are linked to diet alone. The best way to avoid getting cancer is to live a healthy lifestyle and reduce exposure to harmful environmental factors as much as possible. Wear your mask in highly polluted areas, use sunscreens in the sun, limit secondhand exposure to smoking, avoid alcohol consumption, quit smoking, maintain a healthy weight and eat a healthy balanced diet.

We know that preventing disease before it starts is critical to helping us live longer, happier, and healthier lives.

Although chronic diseases are among the costliest of all health problems, they are also among the most preventable.

Proper nutrition can be hard to manage in today's world, especially if you live on the go. Most people don't eat a diet that supplies all the nutrients their body needs.

Vitamins and minerals are an important part of any diet. Even people who eat healthy diets report that taking vitamins increases their energy and improves their health. Supplements are especially useful for people who are unable to get adequate nutrition from their diet alone. Specific conditions, such as gastrointestinal issues, can affect nutrient absorption.

People with restricted diets may also need supplements to ensure they get adequate nutrition. For instance, vegans take vitamin B_{12} since it isn't adequately available in plant foods.

Did you know neuropsychiatric symptoms such as insomnia, depression, anxiety, panic attacks, mania, psychosis, hallucinations, irritability, mood swings, low energy, joint pain, fatigue, and weakness may indicate a vitamin B_{12} deficiency? Taking certain medications can also deplete your vitamin B_{12} levels.

Over 25 percent of people in the United States suffer from these conditions. Ask your doctor to test your vitamin B_{12} levels, and if they are low, consider supplementation. I have helped thousands of my patients support their health and well-being through nutritional deficiency consultations. Since some people do not absorb the tablet formulation due to lack of an intrinsic factor, taking one of the highest-quality isotonic formulations meets the need for B vitamins in a vegetarian diet. Intrinsic factor is a substance naturally found in our gut and is necessary to absorb vitamin B_{12} from the food we eat. Unfortunately, the body sometimes does not make enough intrinsic factor due to certain health conditions and can lead to a type of vitamin B_{12} deficiency known as pernicious anemia. An isotonic formulation of B_{12} contains activated forms of select B vitamins to ensure optimal utilization and quick absorption by the body. Monthly vitamin B_{12} injections are also another option to consider.

If you have any signs or symptoms of chronic fatigue or if you live a high-stress lifestyle, have a weak immune system, take multiple medications, or have hair loss, digestive issues, or thyroid conditions, I highly recommend taking vitamin supplements.

Some supplements interact with prescription medications, and some may not be appropriate for all stages of life, particularly during pregnancy or in breastfeeding women. Some medications such as statins, proton-pump inhibitors, antibiotics, birth control pills, hormone replacement therapy, and even over-the-counter (OTC) products like ibuprofen can deplete important nutrients in your body that need to be replenished.

Every day, I see patients treating themselves with supplements without informing their health care providers. This is appalling as these supplements may interact dangerously with your prescribed medications and may cause serious side effects. Always reach out to your personal pharmacist or to your doctor with any questions you may have before making the purchase.

Since the FDA does not regulate dietary supplements, such as multivitamins, minerals, and herbal supplements, before they go to market, some of these supplements may be contaminated with dangerous ingredients like lead or even pharmaceutical drugs. Many nutritional supplements on retail shelves list ingredients that are not actually in the bottles. You have to always be aware of safety and label accuracy. Know who formulated the product and what their credentials are. A company can claim whatever they want, but without research behind their products, it's likely not the best product to buy.

When choosing a nutritional supplement, you need to take a few more things into consideration. Does the company get every batch tested by an independent third-party researcher? Are their claims true and backed by peer-reviewed research from credible sources like PubMed? Are there studies on their finished product? Most of the time, studies are done to show that individual ingredients are useful, but the real question is whether the final product actually works. The supplements need to be tested, and those results need to be made readily available for the public to read. Also, look at their BBB ratings to verify the integrity and reputation of the company itself.

Most supplements are either based on raw ingredients or synthetic ingredients. "Synthetic" means that the ingredients are sourced from the laboratory. For instance, a synthetic ingredient might be vitamin C from ascorbic acid versus from citrus fruits (its natural form).

When choosing which brands to purchase from, it is important to select supplement brands that provide the purest, highest-quality supplements available. Look for brands with pharmaceutical-grade ingredients. This means that the brands adhere to very rigid manufacturing guidelines. They are made in a current good manufacturing practice, which means a registered manufacturing facility and use of allergen-free ingredients. These products are free of gluten, soy, nuts, fish, dairy, and many other common allergens.

Most popular local retailers and health food stores have supplements that include ingredients that aren't healthy to ingest, such as GMOs, toxic residues, and synthetic food additives. Most retailers leave vitamin supplements sitting for too long on their shelves, which negatively affects their quality as these supplements are supposed to be stored away from heat, light, and humidity. Most drugstores have nutritional products loaded with fillers and synthetic ingredients, and many have little or no active ingredients. These supplement companies are trying to save costs, but the products will only increase your health risks and make you sick.

In fact, tainted supplements send thousands of people to the emergency room every year. Cheaper is not always better. Safety and quality are key.

Look for nutritional companies with the highest-quality supplement brands that frequently sell directly to health care practitioners. I always recommend that patients buy directly from a health care practitioner who is well versed in nutritional products. Ask your health care provider to recommend supplements and drop-ship directly to your mailing address or ask them to direct you to their website to order them yourself. I assist my patients with finding the supplements they need and show them where they can buy them.

It is important to make sure you keep an updated list of all your prescriptions, OTC drugs, vitamin and herbal supplements and have them available to show your pharmacists and other health care providers at every visit.

Pharmacists should make sure there are no drug-drug or drug-supplement interactions and counsel you on how to get the most benefit for your health. They can make sure you are not overdosing on your supplements and that you are not taking what you don't need.

chapter nine

Healthy Movement

Do you work out? A sedentary lifestyle is defined as a type of lifestyle involving little or no physical activity.

According to the WHO, 60 to 85 percent of the population worldwide are not physically active.

Many people drive everywhere they go. This means that they sit in their car to drive to work in the morning, then sit when they get to the office, sit to eat at the cafeteria during their lunch break, sit for office meetings, sit in the car to drive back home for the day, then sit down for dinner and TV until they lay down to sleep, only to repeat this process day after day.

Lifestyle diseases are caused when our genes interact with lifestyle factors that can affect our health and well-being. These include physical inactivity, alcohol, obesity, drugs, poor diet, and smoking.

Getting regular physical activity can help prevent and, in some cases, reverse our risks for lifestyle diseases such as heart disease, obesity, type 2 diabetes, cancer, and high blood pressure.

Moderate exercise can reduce the risk of type 2 diabetes by 50 percent. Another study showed that just one hour of exercise per week can prevent 12 percent of cases of depression. No wonder people are saying that exercise is a natural antidepressant.

Exercise has especially important health benefits for people with chronic conditions. However, it's important to talk to your doctor before starting an exercise routine. Your doctor or health care provider will inform you what exercises are safe and inform you of any cautions you might need to take while exercising to prevent injuries.

Dr. Robert Butler said it best: "If exercise could be purchased in a pill, it would be the single most widely prescribed and beneficial medicine in the nation."

Most health care professionals agree that walking ten thousand steps a day, approximately five miles, is a reasonable target for healthy adults for improving health and reducing the health risks caused by inactivity. It is important to spend quality time outdoors, in nature, every day.

Your busy schedule and unhealthy lifestyle choices can build up your stress levels to cause chronic aches, inflammation, and gut health issues. Therefore, you need to find effective ways to relieve stress. How does the phrase "working out" make you feel? How do you find a form of movement that gets you excited, that you can do as often as you like?

While some people like to work out in groups, like doing Zumba or yoga, to keep their fun and motivation levels high, others look forward to time alone. Some also enjoy spending time working in their garage or in their garden. How can you determine what kinds of exercise will keep you motivated and engaged? One way is to find your fitness style.

Start by experimenting with new exercises that sound fun to you, then choose a few you love and rotate them regularly. Practice them consistently to see which is better suited for you.

The gym industry builds its business model around people not showing up. At the beginning of the year, most people make New Year's resolutions to go to the gym to lose weight and get fit, but how many people actually follow through? Thankfully, there are other effective options than just the gym!

If you haven't been physically fit for a while, you can start today. You can start with light to moderate walking for just five to ten minutes a day. Once you master that, increase the length of your walks until you get to thirty minutes a day of brisk walking, which is where great brain benefits occur.

You can move more and sit less. Think of what you enjoy doing outdoors that will make you happy. Examples are biking, walking, jogging, swimming, dancing, boxing, hiking, climbing, and camping for nature lovers.

Think about playing sports regularly, such as table tennis, soccer, basketball, baseball, softball, or football. You can also just walk up and down the stairs several times a day. Include muscle-strengthening exercises by doing eight reps at least twice a week, such as lifting weights or working with resistance bands. This will help you reduce body fat and increase your muscle mass to help you build healthier, stronger muscles and maintain healthy body weight.

Another thing you can do is keep active at home by mopping the floor regularly, working in your yard or garden, washing your car yourself, and taking long walks on the beach or at the mall.

Park your car further away in the supermarket parking lot, in a safe location, and take every opportunity to walk further to the store.

Stay organized by getting a calendar or a journal and write down your daily exercise schedule. Most people find it easy to start but do not follow through. Make sure to check off each day and time after your exercise. Be consistent.

Ask your family, friends, and even your neighbors to join you. You can encourage them to get healthy with you, and you can hold each other accountable to keep the momentum going.

Regular exercise can increase your mental sharpness and help you focus more. It can increase new brain cells in people of all ages. It is good for your heart. Several studies found that gene expression increases after exercise, causing epigenetic functions to lower the risk of various diseases, including heart disease, obesity, cancer, type 2 diabetes, and high blood pressure.

Rest assured that you can cope with your health challenges using exercise as medicine. If you feel depressed and anxious, go for a walk. If you feel lonely, get out into nature and walk it off. If you are overweight or obese, get up and move around. If you feel stressed out, walk, walk, and keep on walking.

One of the most important things to remember is that your physical activity routine doesn't have to be all or nothing. Take the pressure off to get in a "workout" and simply enjoy moving your body. Try standing up and dancing to songs in your bedroom. It doesn't cost a thing, and you'll feel the benefits right away when you start sweating.

The best thing you can do at any age is to make movement your medicine. We are born for walking.

So with every chance you get during the day, get up and move your body. Remember, do all things in moderation. Wherever you are in your life's journey, just know that it's never too early or too late to start working toward becoming the healthiest you can be. Your body and your future depend on it.

What are you waiting for? Let's get moving!

chapter ten
Restoring Sleep

One in ten people have problems sleeping. We live in a fast-paced world where many people forgo sleep and overextend themselves to catch up on work and other responsibilities. Do you wake up staring at the ceiling? Do you toss and turn in the middle of the night?

When we don't get enough sleep, we wake up feeling tired and irritated, and our diet starts to deteriorate.

There is a direct connection between sleep and health, and it should not be taken lightly.

Sleep can dramatically affect all aspects of our health. Some conditions linked with short sleep duration include chronic pain, cancer, diabetes, hypertension, obesity, heart disease, asthma, GERD, overactive thyroid, Parkinson's disease, and Alzheimer's disease, just to name a few.

The benefits of quality sleep include the following:

- It increases productivity. It gives you the energy to make beneficial lifestyle choices, including choosing to cook healthy meals, deciding to exercise, and taking time for self-care, etc.

- It helps strengthen your immune system, and it builds your body's defenses against infections and chronic health conditions.

- It heightens your alertness, helps you focus, and increases your creativity.

- It improves your mood by reducing anxiety, irritability, and mental exhaustion.

- It increases your sex drive.

- It improves your memory and concentration.

- It reduces stress and lowers your blood pressure.
- It helps you avoid road accidents. It can affect your reaction time as well as decision-making.
- People who sleep well tend to eat fewer calories, while those who lack quality sleep are likely to gain weight over time. They tend to eat more during the day and crave high-fat foods later in the evening.

If you lie in bed for over thirty minutes before being able to fall asleep or wake up in the middle of the night and have trouble falling back asleep most nights of the week, you should think about seeking help because this could mean trouble for you.

If you wake up feeling drained in the morning and have fatigue, headaches, feel depressed, or have memory issues during the daytime multiple times during the week and lasting for three or more months, you should seek medical help.

Every one of us, young and old alike, need optimal sleep for our well-being and optimal health. Try experimenting with your sleep patterns to find out what works best for you and your specific needs.

Are your lifestyle habits causing you sleepless nights? I have had a lot of patients asking for sleep medications, but sleeping pills are not the first solution—getting to the root cause of the problem is. Prescription sleeping pills can be addictive and have side effects such as constipation or diarrhea, difficulty keeping balance, dizziness, daytime drowsiness, dry mouth, and changes in appetite. Also, sleeping pills don't promote restful sleep.

Over-the-counter sleeping pills like Benadryl, Unisom, Tylenol PM, or herbal supplements have side effects as well and can interact dangerously with other medications you're taking and should not be taken long term. Talk to your pharmacist before starting any new drug.

If you are experiencing stress regularly, this can keep you up at night. It can cause you to worry and make you anxious, which will prevent you from falling asleep at night. If you smoke cigarettes frequently and close to bedtime, you will have trouble sleeping at night. If you watch TV late at night, you won't be able to fall asleep. If you play on your phone or work on your computer at night, these devices emit artificial "blue light," which can interfere with your sleep by reducing your melatonin production and keep you awake.

If you find yourself lying in bed for thirty minutes or more and are not able to fall asleep, get up from the bed and do something useful until you feel tired again. Don't stay in bed, and don't expose yourself to blue light by watching TV or browsing the internet.

Only use the bedroom for sleep.

Having a relaxing bedtime routine such as practicing deep breathing, taking a long bath, practicing yoga, listening to relaxing music at a low volume, or being intimate with your spouse may relax you for bedtime.

Choose to limit glutamate-containing foods at night, such as meat, fish, seafood, fermented sauces, and aged cheeses. Eat a variety of healthy foods like quinoa and wild rice, and limit sugar and caffeine intake.

Decide not to overeat close to bedtime because digestion requires energy. When a large meal is eaten at night, it interferes with the body's ability to rest. However, don't go to bed hungry. If you're hungry, try eating a banana or something small instead.

Avoid caffeinated drinks in the evening. Coffee is a stimulant and can keep you up at night. Try not to eat or drink three hours before bedtime. Drinking too much water or other drinks at night can make you go to the bathroom all night long, which disturbs the sleep cycle and hinders sleep quality.

Natural dietary supplements like magnesium, vitamin B_6, and melatonin can support good sleep. Talk to your doctor or pharmacist to find out if they are right for you.

Make sure to have a regular sleep routine schedule. Go to bed at the same time every night. Believe it or not, your body loves to have its own cycle.

Certain medications can interfere with your sleep, so talk to your pharmacist.

Make sure your room is dark at night. Close all the blinds. Feel free to wear an eye mask, headband, or even a scarf wrapped around your eyes at bedtime. Make sure the bedroom temperature is cool and you have a comfortable mattress and a good pillow.

Choose to exercise in the morning or daytime; refrain from exercising close to bedtime.

Stop checking your phones, get off the computer and other devices, and put all electronics away at least one hour before bedtime.

Choose to make your bed every morning when you wake up and declutter your room. It is very important to have a clutter-free space to clear your mind at nighttime. Remember, practice good sleep hygiene habits regularly.

To you all, I say, have a good night.

chapter eleven

The Power of Your Thoughts

Experts estimate that the human mind has, on average, sixty thousand thoughts a day. That's incredible! Are your thoughts mostly positive or negative? Are you the kind of person who normally sees the glass as being half-full or half-empty? I am most grateful for just having a glass of water to drink regardless of the amount.

Scientific studies were done on positive psychology in over forty countries to see what strengths enable people in communities to thrive. Seven characteristics stood out the most as being reliable and well researched. They include expressing gratitude, being optimistic, acts of kindness, using strengths, finding purpose, engaging in empathy, and relishing life in the moment.

Positive emotions are linked to better health, longer life, and greater well-being.

A study showed that rat pups who were loved, cuddled, and nurtured by their mothers had different levels of methylation and different stress responses, which made these rat pups happier and healthier than those abandoned by their mothers. They also showed that these epigenetic effects could be reversed by balancing these deficiencies with loving interventions. Another study showed that women need to be hugged more than once a day to stay healthy. Scientists have shown how a hug a day really keeps the doctor away by increasing the oxytocin levels, which is the love hormone. This is beneficial for our heart health and can lower blood pressure. It can lower cortisol levels, the stress hormone. The good news is that this effect is reciprocal in nature to both the giver as well as the receiver of the hugging. Guys, please hug your women more often. Husbands, when you choose to give your wife more hugs, you're declaring war against life threatening diseases. When you give more hugs, you're shutting down the door to heart disease, heart attack, and helping to lower her blood pressure. When you give more hugs, you're insulating your wife's body from the harmful effects of stress throughout the day. When you give hugs, you're restoring your wife's body back to health. When you give your wife more hugs, you're choosing to give her the body she wants.

We all need more hugs. Let's get in the habit of giving more hugs as the benefits are reciprocal—you get it right back! Let's all do our part to combat chronic health conditions, loneliness, anxiety, depression and touch the souls of men, women, youth, and children by dispensing more hugs. Let it start today and let it start with you.

Could early childhood care in humans also affect methylation levels?

Scientists discovered important differences between the brains of suicide victims and people with normal brains who died from other causes. There was a link between certain epigenetic patterns, suicide, and child abuse.

All thirteen suicide victims in the study had experienced abuse as children. The scientists were especially interested in a part of the brain called the hippocampus, which is involved in learning, memory, and mood. This area of the brain was found to be smaller in people who had suffered abuse growing up.

They inspected genes in the hippocampus involved in controlling protein-producing RNA and interestingly found that in the suicide victims a much higher proportion of these genes had been switched off, meaning that the hippocampus was less active.

Your subconscious mind cannot tell the difference between a real event and something you just thought about.

Have you ever woken up from a nightmare shaking uncontrollably and feeling scared to get out of bed?

Recently, I had a very bad dream about my father, where everyone was crying, and I woke up with real tears on my face. My heart was still pounding, my whole body was physically shaking, and sweat dripped down my forehead. Even though I wasn't in real danger when I woke up from that bad dream, I was experiencing all the psychological reactions in my body physically. My fear-based thoughts activated my hypothalamus, which activated my endocrine system and caused my adrenal glands to produce more cortisol, the stress hormone. The dream was so vivid that I decided to call my dad as soon as it was daylight outside, just to make sure he was okay as he lived in another state. Thank God, he was fine then. Unfortunately, my dad died the very next day. No sickness, no hurting, no pain. The doctor said he died of natural causes. Although, it's been three years now, the physical pain still felt like it was yesterday. I miss our talks, and I miss his presence, his advice, his encouragement, his prayers, his support, and, most importantly, his unconditional love. I just miss you so much, Dad. What a great loss! Your legacy lives on. Continue to rest in peace till we meet again, Dad. I can't wait till resurrection morning to be reunited with you.

Through it all, I was reminded that tomorrow is not promised to us, and there's no time to waste. I choose to find my purpose on earth. It took a lot to get here, to be present every moment to self-improve and grow to become the best version of me. I am intentional in my daily actions to help others with my knowledge and to give back to my community. I am choosing to give encouragement and hope to someone who sees no way out. I am choosing to make a friend smile even though she's hit rock bottom. I am choosing to actively listen to my patients to best help them get to the root cause and find practical solutions to improve their health outcomes. I am choosing to educate patients and their families about chronic health conditions and to connect them with clinical services and appropriate community resources. I am choosing to make this world a better place, one person at a time, one day at a time, and one kind act at a time. Do you know your purpose? Why are you here on earth? How do you deal with difficult situations or tragedies?

Your thoughts can influence your health and weaken your immune system. Your thoughts can cause anxiety by worrying too much about things you can't change. What you see, smell, hear, and taste can all shape your unconscious mind.

The mind plays a critical role in the perception of pain. Alia Crum, a clinical psychologist, shows in her research that those who expect worse pain and dwell on it feel more intense pain, stay longer in hospitals after surgery, and often require more pain medication. Likewise, those who shift to a positive mindset feel less pain, spend less time in hospitals, and require fewer pain medications.

Another study from John Hopkins University found that people with a family history of heart disease, even in those with the most risk factors for coronary artery disease, who also had a positive outlook were one-third less likely to have a heart attack or other cardiovascular event within five to twenty-five years than those with a more negative outlook.

Our minds can actually change our reality. You can use what you think about and how you are thinking to improve your epigenetics. If you can heal your mind, you can also heal your body.

You can learn how to flip negative thoughts to positive thoughts to activate your endorphins to produce good feelings.

To start controlling your thoughts, start with the first thoughts of the day. Do all you can to make sure your first thoughts of the day are love- based. When you get up in the morning, start by monitoring your thoughts and then start flipping them to what you want them to be.

Another thing you can do is practice being thankful throughout the day. Start every day with a heartfelt prayer of thanksgiving. Spend your time thinking about things you are thankful for. When you get upset, show appreciation for something that happened to you earlier in the day. Choose to dwell on the positive things and ignore the negative ones. Give yourself permission to smile or laugh more. Watch funny videos. Practice positive thinking every day. Choose to be in control of your thoughts.

Conclusion

"**M**ind your thoughts." Your thoughts can affect your reality and everything that happens to you in life. When you actively invest your attention into your thoughts, they begin to seem real. They can become your words and lead to certain actions, which can form certain lifestyle habits and lead to character traits and what you eventually become in life. In other words, you can basically focus on success and attract success, and the same is also true if you focus on fear and failure.

Most people make a New Year's resolution at the beginning of every year, but why not make a new day resolution every day about improving your lifestyle habits? Why not ask the Holy Spirit to lead and guide everything you do in life including your lifestyle choices so that you can make decisions within the blueprint of God's will?

For I know the plans I have for you, declares the Lord, plans to prosper you and not to harm you, plans to give you hope and a future.
—Jeremiah 29:11

There is power in spoken words. Repeat these affirmations every morning before you get out of bed. The only caveat here is that you have to believe in what you are saying. Believe it from your heart and confess it with your mouth. Power is being released into the atmosphere by what you say. Speak life into your situations every day. Speak blessings and you shall have what you desire. All things are possible if only you believe. Go ahead and say them out loud now:

"I am taking deep breaths to lower stress in my body."
"I am loving myself unconditionally, and I forgive myself."
"I am letting go of what does not serve me any longer."
"I am an overcomer. I am a fighter. I am a survivor."
"I am letting go of all my past childhood traumas."
"I am letting go of the sickness and pain that are weighing me down."

"I am letting go of all excuses and will start taking charge of my own health."

"I am grateful for my healthy body."

"I am healed deep down in my heart."

Start each new day by evaluating where you are now in your health journey. How did you get here? What have you learned from your experiences? Are you still following the same lifestyle habits that got you here? Are you growing and learning to improve your health? Are you stuck in your pain, sickness, negative thoughts, bitterness, or hatred?

Life happens to all of us, so what's your story?

We learned how damaging childhood traumas can affect us for life. How much are you still hurting from the past? How long will you continue to dwell on how someone you love dealt with you so unfairly? Life is not fair, but you don't have to live in the past actions of others. When you feel stuck, choose to move forward; never go backward. It's never too late to start over again regardless of your age or wherever you are in your life's journey. You can choose to believe that your past no longer defines you. Learn from your past mistakes, break the chains, and choose to open the door to a brighter future.

Are you ready to forgive those who hurt you badly in the past so that your body can begin to heal itself? Are you choosing to continue to harbor hate and resentment in your heart? That burden is too big to carry throughout your life. Choose to forgive and let it go. Forgive and forget so you can grow. Forgive so you can clear your mind of all the unnecessary burdens that are damaging your body. Allow your heart to heal. I know it's not easy to forgive and forget. I know the pain is real. I know a pill isn't strong enough to reach this level of a broken heart. However, to be healthy, you must choose to let it go now. It's time to unload all the baggage. Cry if you must, but forgive for your own good, for your health's sake, for the sake of your loved ones, and for the future generations.

Declare war against every sickness in your body, against pain, against past childhood traumas, against negative thoughts.

Activate your mind with healing powers. You are in charge now. Talk to your health issues with the authority you have inside of your body. Repeat these words: "I am standing up for my health. The hurt I experienced was then; my healing is now. I am no longer afraid of history repeating itself in the future. I release every negative thought, guilt, and revenge that are holding me back from healing. I am breaking the chain of sickness, breaking the chain of worry, breaking the chain of negative thoughts bombarding my mind."

Start reinventing your health. Repeat: "I was used to sitting down all the time. That's what I used to do in the past. I am improving my daily habits now. If I knew better, I would've done better. I am getting up every thirty minutes to move more. I am cutting down on sugary drinks now. I am stopping the cigars. I am letting go of my negative mindset. I am starting to eat clean. I am forgiving myself unconditionally. I am deciding to start losing some weight. I am giving my body the sleep it needs. I am letting go of toxic relationships. I am enforcing boundaries and going with my standards. I am getting clear on my priorities and becoming more intentional. I am getting the help I need by talking and working through my problems." It is through the small victories in maintaining our emotional health that we gain the self confidence that we need to fight.

Take full responsibility and accept where you are now in your health journey. Take the responsibility to change your poor health outcome. Not your doctor, not your pharmacist, not the nurse, but you. Only you are in charge of your own health. Own that responsibility. Repeat:

"I will run five miles every morning, starting at 6:15 a.m."

"I will eat fruits and vegetables along with every meal. I will regularly remind myself to throw away all the junk foods in my pantry and replace them with healthy options."

"I will take deep breaths and calm down whenever I feel angry. I will take the necessary steps to control my stress."

Are things very bad right now with your health issues? Maybe you don't see a way out, and your doctor has run out of options. Maybe your pain is unbearable, and your health situation seems hopeless. If you're struggling with health issues and reading this now, I pray you find the strength and the courage to keep fighting for your health. You're almost there! Healing is coming. Hold on. Remember, your current situation is not permanent.

This too shall pass. Don't quit. Don't you dare give up now. Suicide is not an option!

Repeat: "I expect things to get better for me. I am improving and getting better and healthier. My problems are temporary. As long as I have breath in me, it's not the end. Things can only go up from here on. My body is receiving healing in abundance."

Take positive actions toward your health.

Get up and go for a walk.

Pick up an inspiring book and start reading chapter 1 today.

Listen to uplifting songs.

Stay busy to take your mind off your pain and suffering.

Help somebody else when you feel like giving up on yourself. Encourage someone, even when you are down in spirit. Give thanks and appreciation for your life. Be grateful for what you have now, and always keep hope alive.

Change your current strategies and start over from here. Invest in a health coach. Find somebody who loves you and cares about you, somebody who will hold you accountable to help you reach your health goals. Somebody who will support you and be your cheerleader. We all could use a little help.

Do you know what your body needs to stay healthy? Do you know what your body wants?

Join me in creating a movement to combat chronic health issues through healthy lifestyle changes. Together, we can make this world a healthier place.

Remember, God loves you and so do I. I wish you all the best of health.

Beloved, I pray that you may prosper in all things and be in health, just as your soul prospers.

—3 John 2

Acknowledgments

In loving memory of Daniel Oshundele, my beloved dad who raised me to always be giving. He is a model of compassion who has driven my passion to help people, which led me to my interest in health care.

And as always, I am grateful to my children, Chukey and Chuka Wachuku, for their steadfast patience and kindness, for always cheering me on to continue to write, and for never complaining about not spending that time with them.

I also want to thank my mom, Esther Oshundele, for her continued love, prayers, and support.

I want to thank my siblings Eunice Oshundele, Dorcas Oyebanji, Grace Dada, Maria McErleane, and Segun Osundele for their love and encouragement.

I also want to thank my sisters-in-law, Adanna Izeko and Cassandra Osundele, for their advice and insight.

And what a great pleasure to work with Emily Nutter, my editor. Thanks so much for editing my book and doing an awesome job. I am very grateful.

Above all, I thank the Almighty God for sparing my life to see this day.

About the Author

Dr. Christina Wachuku graduated from Long Island University in New York with a degree in pharmacology (Doctor of Pharmacy; PharmD). She is an independent consultant pharmacist, medical information pharmacist specialist, and an integrative nutrition health coach, board certified in ambulatory care pharmacy and antiaging medicine.

She conducts private consultations with her clientele to help them better understand the purpose of their medications and how to use them appropriately to curb adverse drug reactions, reduce medication risks, and identify ways to increase savings in costs of medications. She is committed to helping those trying to lose weight keep it off with healthy habits that are scientifically based and unique to their lifestyle. She works to improve her patients' health with personalized plans through education, encouragement, accountability, and support.

She became a credentialed provider with the military and helped implement MTM services into their clinic. She is certified as a pharmacist genetic drug counselor.

She continually goes for continuing education unit and attends conferences and workshops where she has received over one hundred contact hours of continuing education every year. She is also an active subscriber to pharmacy journals such as *Pharmacy Today* and *US Pharmacist* to keep up on current guidelines on primary works of literature. She uses this knowledge to help improve her patients' lives in her day-to-day interactions with them. This helps her keep up to date with the ever-changing guidelines and new innovative scientific-based practices.

MediFixx Health, LLC, is the brainchild that she established to help patients at increased risk of morbidity and mortality due to medication-related problems. She aims to make a measurable impact that will transform their lives through personalized one-on-one consultation services and improve their health outcomes.

References

1. Centers for Disease Control and Prevention. "Adverse Childhood Experiences Reported by Adults—Five States." *Morbidity and Mortality Weekly Report* 59, no. 49 (2009): 1609–13.

2. Department of Health and Human Services. *Summary Health Statistics for the U.S. Population: National Health Interview Survey 2012.* http://www.cdc.gov/nchs/data/series/sr_10/sr10_259.pdf.

3. Derbyshire, David. "Loneliness Is a Killer: It's as Bad for Your Health as Alcoholism, Smoking, and Over-Eating, Say Scientists." Health Mail Online, last modified Dec 2021. https://www.researchgate.net/publication/333425627_Loneliness_Matters_A_Theoretical_Review_of_Prevalence_in_Adulthood/citation/download

4. Kaati, G., L. O. Bygren, and S. Edvinsson. "Cardiovascular and Diabetes Mortality Determined by Nutrition during Parents' and Grandparents' Slow Growth Period." *European Journal of Human Genetics* 10, no. 11 (2002): 682–8. https://doi.org/10.1038/sj.ejhg.5200859.

5. Kolonel, L. N., D. Altshuler, and B. E. Henderson. "The Multiethnic Cohort Study: Exploring Genes, Lifestyle and Cancer Risk." *Nat Rev Cancer* 4 (2004): 519–27. https://doi.org/10.1038/nrc1389

6. Fraga, Mario F., Esteban Baluster, Maria F. Paz, Santiago Ropero, Fernando Setien, Maria L. Ballestar, Damia Heine-Suner, et al. "Epigenetic Differences Arise during the Lifetime of Monozygotic Twins." *PNAS* 102, no. 30 (2005): 10604–9. https://doi.org/10.1073/pnas.0500398102.

7. Metzler, Marilyn, Melissa T. Merrick, Joanne Klevens, Katie A. Ports, and Derek C. Ford. "Adverse Childhood Experiences and Life Opportunities: Shifting the Narrative." *Children and Youth Services Review* 72 (2017): 141–9. https://doi.org/10.1016/j.childyouth.2016.10.021.

8. Mocchegiani, E., L. Costarelli, R. Giacconi, et al., "Vitamin E-Gene Interactions in Aging and Inflammatory Age-Related Diseases: Implications for Treatment. A Systematic Review." *Ageing Research Reviews* 14 (2014): 81–101.

9. Metzler, M., M. T. Merrick, J. Klevens, K. A. Ports, and D. C. Ford. "Adverse Childhood Experiences and Life Opportunities: Shifting the Narrative." *Children and Youth Services Review* 72 (2017): 141–9.

10. National Center for Chronic Disease Prevention and Health Promotion. "The Power of Prevention." Centers for Disease Control and Prevention. http://www.cdc.gov/chronicdisease/pdf/2009-Power-of-Prevention.pdf.

11. National Center for Health Statistics. "Summary Health Statistics for the U.S. Population: National Health Interview Survey, 2012." Centers for Disease Control and Prevention, 2013.

12. P. Irigaray, J. A. Newby, R. Clapp, L. Hardell, V. Howard, L. Montagnier, S. Epstein, and D. Belpomme. Lifestyle-related factors and environmental agents causing cancer: an overview. Biomed. Pharmacother.61:640–58 (2007) doi:10.1016/j.biopha.2007.10.006. [PubMed]

13. Prüss-Üstün, Annette C. C. "Preventing Disease through Healthy Environments. Towards an Estimate of the Environmental Burden of Disease." World Health Organization, 2006.

14. Stravynski, A., and R. Boyer. "Loneliness in Relation to Suicide Ideation and Parasuicide: A Population-Wide Study." *Suicide Life Threat Behavior* 31, no. 1 (2001): 32–40. https://doi.org/10.1521/suli.31.1.32.21312.

15. "Tackling the Burden of Chronic Diseases in the USA." *The Lancet* 373, no 9659 (2009): 185. https://doi.org/10.1016/S0140-6736(09)60048-9.

16. Tsancova N, Renthal W, Kumar A, and Nextler E. J. "Epigenetic Regulation in Psychiatric Disorders." *Nature Reviews Neuroscience* 8 (2007): 355–67.

17. Vinje, S., E. Stroes, M. Nieuwdorp, et al. "The Gut Microbiome as Novel Cardiometabolic Target: The Time Has Come!" *Eur Heart J* 35 (2014): 883–7.

18. Wilson, Robert S., Kristin R. Krueger, Steven E. Arnold, Julie A. Schneider, Jeremiah F. Kelly, Lisa L. Barnes, Yuxiao Tang, et al. "Loneliness and Risk of Alzheimer Disease." *Arch Gen Psychiatry* 64, no. 2 (2007): 234–240. https://doi.org/10.1001/archpsyc.64.2.234.

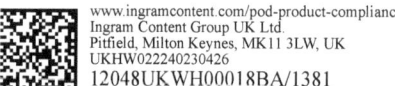
www.ingramcontent.com/pod-product-compliance
Ingram Content Group UK Ltd.
Pitfield, Milton Keynes, MK11 3LW, UK
UKHW022240230426
12048UKWH00018BA/1381